Uncover Abundant New Sources of Power

Each of us is endowed with the energies of life and the powers of personal consciousness. By living younger, longer, and better, we can learn new approaches for achieving our goals, overcoming obstacles, conquering adversity, and living a more productive life. By keeping our minds youthful, creative, and dynamic, we can find more effective ways of acquiring new knowledge, discovering our inner landscape, re-energizing the mind, and finally realizing our highest potentials. In a word, we can become *empowered*. Having achieved personal empowerment, we can, in turn, create a better world for ourselves and our children. . . .

The rejuvenation strategies presented in this book are structured to uncover abundant new sources of power, both within ourselves and beyond. Through our rejuvenation efforts, we discover that we can take command of our lives and the forces that affect our existence. We discover that we can set goals and achieve them. Even more important, we discover that we can determine our ultimate destiny.

About the Author

Joe H. Slate, Ph.D. (Alabama), is a licensed psychologist, professor, and founder of the International Parapsychology Research Foundation. He has appeared on numerous talk shows and television programs, including *Sightings* and *Strange Universe*.

To Write to the Author

If you wish to contact the author or would like more information about this book, please write to the author in care of Llewellyn Worldwide and we will forward your request. Both the author and publisher appreciate hearing from you and learning of your enjoyment of this book and how it has helped you. Llewellyn Worldwide cannot guarantee that every letter written to the author can be answered, but all will be forwarded. Please write to:

Joe H. Slate
℅ Llewellyn Worldwide
P.O. Box 64383, Dept. 1-56718-633-5
St. Paul, MN 55164-0383, U.S.A.

Please enclose a self-addressed stamped envelope for reply,
or $1.00 to cover costs. If outside U.S.A., enclose
international postal reply coupon.

Many of Llewellyn's authors have websites with additional information and resources. For more information, please visit our website at www.llewellyn.com.

JOE H. SLATE, Ph.D.

REJUVENATION

Strategies for Living Younger, Longer & Better

Includes CD and 7-Day Plan

2001
Llewellyn Publications
St. Paul, Minnesota 55164-0383, U.S.A.

First Edition
First Printing, 2001

Book design and editing by Michael Maupin
Cover design by Lisa Novak

Library of Congress Cataloging-in-Publication Data
Slate, Joe H.
    Rejuvenation : strategies for living younger, longer & better / Joe H. Slate.
        p.   cm.
    Includes bibliographical references and index.
    ISBN 1-56718-633-5
    1. Rejuvenation. 2. Longevity. 3. Aging—Prevention. I. Title.

RA777.6 .S595 2001
613—dc21   00-067006

Llewellyn Worldwide does not participate in, endorse, or have any authority or responsibility concerning private business transactions between our authors and the public.

All mail addressed to the author is forwarded but the publisher cannot, unless specifically instructed by the author, give out an address or phone number.

Any Internet references contained in this work are current at publication time, but the publisher cannot guarantee that a specific location will continue to be maintained. Please refer to the publisher's website for links to authors' websites and other sources.

Note: The practices, techniques, and meditations described in this book should not be used as an alternative to professional medical treatment. This book does not attempt to give any medical diagnosis, treatment, prescription, or suggestion for medication in relation to any human disease, pain, injury, deformity, or physical condition.

The author and publisher of this book are not responsible in any manner whatsoever for any injury which may occur through following the instructions contained herein. It is recommended that before beginning any alternative healing practice you consult with your physician to determine whether you are medically, physically, and mentally fit to undertake the practice.

The CD included with this book should be used only under safe, controlled conditions. It should not be used under conditions requiring alertness and vigilance, such as while driving or operating machinery.

Llewellyn Publications
A Division of Llewellyn Worldwide, Ltd.
P.O. Box 64383, Dept. 1-56718-633-5
St. Paul, MN 55164-0383, U.S.A.
www.llewellyn.com

Printed in the United States of America

Other Books by Joe H. Slate

Psychic Empowerment

Psychic Empowerment for Health and Fitness

Astral Projection and Psychic Empowerment

Aura Energy for Health, Healing & Balance

Contents

Author's Notes ix
Preface xi

Author's Notes

As professor of psychology at Athens State College (now Athens State University), I taught life-span psychology for several years, during which time I became increasingly aware that the aging process is fluid rather than fixed. It became more and more obvious that many of the major factors that influence the rate of aging are neither absolute nor immutable, but instead flexible and responsive to our deliberate intervention. We can redirect them and alter their effects on the mind and body. Identifying the elements that promote rejuvenation and longevity as well as the quality of life became one of my major interests and the topic of numerous research efforts which provided the empirical basis for many of the strategies presented in this book.

To the students who participated in my life-span studies, I wish to express my sincerest appreciation. Some of them helped conduct interviews, field studies, and surveys which yielded critical data on rejuvenation and longevity. Other students became laboratory assistants whose insights and skills contributed immeasurable to the development of structured procedures ranging from the use of altered states to tangible objects as rejuvenation tools. I will be forever indebted to all of them for enthusiastically giving of their time and energy in the search for new understanding of rejuvenation and longevity.

To the scores of experimental subjects who volunteered to participate in my research efforts, I wish to express my heartfelt thanks. Without their participation, this project could not have been completed.

To my learned colleagues who contributed their ideas and offered both advice and criticism for the duration of this effort, I also wish to express my sincerest thanks. I wish to express special thanks to two former presidents of Athens State University, Dr. Frank Philpot and Dr. Sidney Sandridge, for their encouragement and support of my work. Both men, who themselves seemed to have conquered aging, were a source of inspiration from the earliest beginnings of my research on rejuvenation. I will be forever indebted to them. I am also grateful to Dr. Clark Schmidt, president of Celestial Visions of Metaphysical Arts, for his insightful suggestions and contributions to this effort. I wish also to thank Bryan Forbes of Slate Security Systems, Inc. for his invaluable technical advice and assistance.

Finally, to the men and women at Llewellyn Publications, I here express my sincerest thanks for their continuing encouragement and interest in my work.

PREFACE

The constant focus of this book is on living younger, longer, and better. Because of the many new breakthroughs in our understanding of rejuvenation, we can finally discard the old adage, "To age too soon, to learn too late." It is never too late to learn new, exciting ways of living younger, longer, and better. Although nature may have dealt the biological cards, it's up to us to play them. We can now take command of the game.

Rejuvenation by definition is the process of making young or youthful by restoring or renewing anti-aging powers. As an emerging new technology, rejuvenation is a combination of art and science which brings together *quality* and *quantity* of life as never before. As an art, it offers creative strategies and practical procedures designed to activate the rejuvenation process and maximize its capacity to enrich our lives. As a science, it is an evolving body of knowledge based of years of research, much of it in the highly controlled laboratory setting.

Successful rejuvenation, like self-empowerment, is a continuous, developmental phenomenon which is as refined as each element it entails. It beckons each of us with its promise of a richer, happier, and more fulfilled life. It sets a new standard for living each day with quality and extraordinary, incredible joy.

At last, the luxurious pleasures of rejuvenation are within your reach. Senescence is no longer your irremediable destiny. You can jump-start the rejuvenation process and turbocharge your inner age-defying mechanisms. All it takes is a workable plan and a basic passion for change. That's why the rejuvenation procedures presented in this book stipulate a sleek combination of specific goals and unyielding motivation.

According to an old Taoist saying, "The journey is the reward." Starting now, you can get on the expressway to rejuvenation. Even better, you can write your own ticket and punch it too.

CHAPTER 1

Rejuvenation and the Energies of Life

Our existence in the universe can be described in many ways, but nothing comes closer to the mark than the simple fact that we are an *energy force*. Whether we spring from an energized mix of cosmic dust that eventually spawned life, or from a sudden stroke of infinite power, we all share a single fountainhead of energy, without which we would not exist. Scripturally speaking, *He hath made of one blood (energy) all men to dwell on the face of the earth*. Moreover, we share a common need—to understand our place in the universe and to realize our highest potentials for growth and fulfillment. Only then can we experience the magnificence of our personal existence and the splendor of the collective cosmos of which we are an integral part.

Given the cosmic nature of our origin, it requires no quantum leap to acknowledge the invincible, indestructible nature of our being. As an infinite life force, we are temporary residents of the planet, but permanent citizens of the immeasurable cosmos with full access to its inexhaustible resources. We, like the dynamic

1

energies that sustain the universe itself, are a perpetual force within a higher cosmic scheme. Rather than *possessing* energy, we *are* energy. It is the essence of our existence. It is the life force unique to each of us. It is the architectural design through which our existence—mentally, physically, and spiritually—finds purpose and identity. Its evolution throughout our lifetimes enables us to explore options, accommodate change, create new possibilities, and initiate new growth—in other words, to achieve our highest destiny for greatness.

One view of human existence holds that we have a predetermined amount of energy to expend in a given lifetime. Once that energy supply is exhausted, our existence in that lifetime expires. According to this view, some individuals are endowed with a minimal energy supply, which is typically expended over a brief lifetime, whereas others possess an abundant energy supply sustaining them over a long lifetime. Future lifetimes would require additional appropriations of energy, the amount of which would be based on predetermined lifetime goals, and the time and energy required to achieve them. Although this view implies predestination, it emphasizes that too much of our energy expenditure is wasteful and inefficient. It holds that our existence in a given lifetime can be thwarted and even cut short on the one hand, or it can be extended and enriched through deliberate intervention and mastery of appropriate energy conservation and use strategies.

Another view of human existence holds that each of us is endowed with inexhaustible potential to create abundant energy. But according to this view, unlimited potential does not necessarily translate into an unlimited supply of available energy. The internal energy system must be developed and maintained. Efficient energy production and conservation strategies must be acquired, and effective techniques for using energy must be mastered.

Common to both of the above views is the human capacity for intervention and control. The belief that we can do little or nothing to arrest aging and reverse its effects is profoundly pessimistic and, fortunately, wrong. It's like saying we can do little or nothing to protect and nurture our environment. Like our global survival, our personal well-being demands decisive action. Beyond diet, exercise, and appropriate medical care, we can master new strategies that prolong life and repair time's damages.

Even from a purely economic perspective, living longer and staying healthy have important implications. Ironically, in our culture, dying young is more expensive than dying old. Incredible as it may seem, the health care costs during their last two years of life for seventy-year-olds is more than twice that for centenarians. This remarkable phenomenon implies that centenarians may have discovered for themselves many of the secrets for a longer, healthier life. It comes as no surprise then that scientists have studied centenarians for years in an attempt to uncover their secrets. Some of the rejuvenation procedures discussed in this book are, in fact, based on our studies of centenarians. By maximizing their rejuvenation powers, many centenarians seemed to find ways of preventing costly illnesses that commonly come with aging. A major goal of rejuvenation is to avoid living through years of chronic disease and dependence before death.

The forty-five rejuvenation strategies presented in the following chapters are based on the simple premise that, rather than becoming a globe in the grips of aging, we can slow the winged chariot of time and live a longer, richer life. Preventing genetic mutations that cause illness, keeping artery walls open and free of blockage, and prolonging the ability of cells to reproduce are reasonable expectations for all who are willing to develop their capacities for rejuvenation and longevity.

According to conventional wisdom, our genetic limit for longevity is around 100 years. But most people do not achieve that potential. This may be due to our perceptions of aging, and a tendency to become less active mentally and physically as we grow in years. A more vicious factor is the not-so-subtle cultural expectation that we *must* age, that there is little or nothing we can do about it. Furthermore, as we age, we *must* take on the characteristics expected of the aged. We are expected to yield to the indignities of *ageism,* a common stereotype in our culture. Being older is alone often sufficient to result in a dramatic downward shift in status and recognition. When accompanied by retirement, the shift can be particularly acute. We are culturally conditioned to see no option but to submit to the inevitable, irreversible effects of aging. In the worst scenario, we become like sheep led to the slaughter, passive victims of overwhelming forces that seem beyond our control.

On a massive scale, we may have contributed to cultural stereotypes of aging by unconsciously programming our own physical body at an early age to meet cultural life-span expectations. In the next century, we will probably look back on this incredible practice with amazement. Mark Twain offers a familiar example of the expectancy effect of targeting one's own death. Born at the appearance of Halley's comet, he accurately predicted his death—and unfortunately programmed himself for it—at the comet's re-appearance. Further supporting the expectancy effects on longevity is the postponement of death as sometimes seen among the terminally ill. Consciously or subconsciously, they often delay death until after a significant life event, such as an anniversary or holiday. These observations suggest that we can deliberately take command of both life and death. A strong internal energy system, along with mastery of new rejuvenation and longevity skills, could equip us to control aging and determine our life's destiny.

Among the essential conditions for developing a powerful energy system are a positive self-concept and a keen sense of personal worth. But even with these elements in place, we are often bombarded by negative forces that threaten our growth and exact a heavy toll on our total well-being. Examples of these forces include the wear-and-tear of long-term stress, the pressures of daily life, unresolved personal conflicts, and severe crises, such as the death of a loved one, breakup of a relationship, serious illness, unemployment, and financial reversal—all of which can literally alter the direction and pace of our growth—mentally, physically, and spiritually.

Additional influences affecting the human energy system are our interactions with others. As a general rule, positive interactions generate positive energy that promotes our personal well-being, whereas negative interactions rapidly deplete our supply of positive energy. This cardinal principle applies not only to person-to-person and group-to-group interactions, it is valid on an international scale. Interactions among nations that recognize human worth create a critical force that can infuse the globe with positive energy. It would follow that global peace must eventually flow, not from the massive destruction of war, but form positive energy generated on a global scale. At a very practical level, the energies and resources consumed by war, if expended on peace, would make the globe a safer, richer, and healthier place for everyone. The money spent on weapons alone could eradicate global hunger and poverty. We owe it to ourselves and the children of the world to end once and for all the atrocities of war.

Successful Rejuvenation and Personal Empowerment

Each of us is endowed with the energies of life and the powers of personal consciousness. By living younger, longer, and better, we can learn new approaches for achieving our goals, overcoming obstacles, conquering adversity, and living a more productive life. By keeping our minds youthful, creative, and dynamic, we can find more effective ways of acquiring new knowledge, discovering our inner landscape, re-energizing the mind, and finally realizing our highest potentials. In a word, we can become *empowered*. Having achieved personal empowerment, we can, in turn, create a better world for ourselves and our children.

But in the real world, our struggle to achieve our noblest goals often gets interrupted and our strivings become thwarted. We lose sight of our strengths and give in to our weaknesses. We succumb to discouragement, and all too often, we lose faith in ourselves and our hope for the future.

The rejuvenation strategies presented in this book are structured to uncover abundant, new sources of power, both within ourselves and beyond. Through our rejuvenation efforts, we discover that we can take command of our lives and the forces that affect our existence. We discover that we can set goals and achieve them. Even more important, we discover that we can determine our ultimate destiny.

Finding new ways of living longer, younger, and better will be part of the big challenges facing us as we enter the new millennium. We know, of course, that we can promote personal fitness through a healthful lifestyle that includes proper exercise and nutrition. But we can't afford to stop there. We must find ways of complementing these basics with solid anti-aging strategies that effectively rejuvenate the mind, body, and spirit. At an even higher level, we must master the complex mechanisms that fuel the aging process itself.

A simplistic view of human existence focuses on aging as simply a natural, biological phenomenon which, for the most part, is autonomous and thus beyond our conscious control. This view either minimizes or overlooks altogether the critical mental and spiritual components of the aging process. In contrast, the personal empowerment perspective on aging, while recognizing crucial biological influences, emphasizes the human capacity to deliberately intervene to alter the aging process and the underlying components that energize it. This perspective recognizes the effects of excessive stress, depression, hopelessness, and a poor self-image—all of which accelerate aging by depleting our reserve of positive energy. It recognizes the power of spiritual insight, to include a sharp awareness of our high place in the universe. It emphasizes our capacity to interact with our biological makeup and self-system in ways that rejuvenate the physical body and improve the total quality of our existence. It holds unequivocally that we can deliberately take command of all negative components that accelerate aging. As a result, the quality of our lives is enhanced, the aging process is slowed, and in many instances, the effects of aging on both the mind and body are literally eradicated. Rather than surrendering to the aging process, we find ways of subduing and defeating it. Among the aims of this book is to identify age accelerants and formulate procedures that eliminate them.

As human beings, we are designed to grow, not deteriorate. The physical body seeks youth and health. It is always responsive to our efforts to stay young and undo aging. Rejuvenation is a natural process of renewal and growth. We have the built-in potential to repair, re-create, and rejuvenate ourselves. By developing that potential, we could conceivably live and grow indefinitely while, at the same time, improving the quality of our existence. But all too often, we reject the sources of rejuvenation within ourselves and our surroundings. As a result, our biological systems slowly deteriorate, and our bodies finally wear out—all within an artificially fixed life span that we accept as absolute and immutable. Because we expect to age and die, we eventually self-destruct. We fail to discover the limitless possibilities for continued growth and fulfillment.

A major focus of this book is on self-determination and self-empowerment. We cannot afford to wait for science to provide some magic rejuvenation formula. Although an effective "rejuvenation pill" may eventually become available, we already know enough about rejuvenation and longevity to take the initiative in

determining our life span. A host of innovative anti-aging strategies, many of them developed in our laboratory or uncovered in
our field studies, are now available to everyone. With mastery of
this emerging technology, much of it focusing on the sheer
power of the human mind and spirit, we can each become
empowered to choose how long to live in this lifetime; and even
more important than that, we can constantly improve the richness of our existence.

Although injury, disease, and suffering are realistically a part
of life, none of them can shatter the empowered spirit. We can
learn from them, and then push forward with even greater purpose, quality, and power. Eventually, of course, death will lean
against the door, but rather than prolonged chronic illness, we
can experience a smooth, joyous passage to the other side. We
can make our exit from this dimension, not with whimpering
defeat, but with triumphant celebration. Death, having been
"swallowed up in victory," becomes a wondrous transition that
crowns our growth in one dimension, while opening the gateway for endless growth in another.

The Golden Rules of Rejuvenation

Whatever our age, and wherever we are in our personal growth,
certain golden rules are relevant to all our rejuvenation efforts.
Each rule is built on the belief that quality existence is the
birthright of every individual. But achieving that empowered
state requires effort and determination. By embracing each of
the following principles, we can maximize our potentials, not
only for successful rejuvenation, but also for an enriched,
empowered life.

> **Rule 1. Discover the supreme power of your mind.**
> Your physical body with its multiple processes, includ-
> ing the mechanisms of aging, is responsive to the
> powers of your mind. Even the body's so-called auto-

nomic functions are subservient to the mind. Use your mind to listen to your body. Become quiet and attentive to what you body is telling you.

Rule 2. Recognize the cosmic nature of your existence. When you plug into your cosmic origins, you become the sole master of your life. Many of the strategies presented in this book are structured either to activate your inner cosmic resources or to access higher cosmic powers.

Rule 3. Acknowledge your worth and the worth of others. This is one of the most important enabling values known. Only when we accept our own worth can we accept the worth of others. Recognizing the incomparable value of yourself and others is a critical focal point for successful rejuvenation.

Rule 4. Establish strong bonds of family, friends, and faith. They will sustain you through the good times and the bad. Faith and the social support of family and friends are universally empowering.

Rule 5. Identify your rejuvenation goals and commit yourself to them. Establish clear, positive goals that involve not only a good diet and exercise, but the innermost part of yourself as well. The single greatest reason that rejuvenation efforts fail is a tendency to view them as physical goals only. By setting deeply meaningful goals, taking decisive action to achieve them, and persisting without wavering, you will succeed.

Rule 6. Recognize the interactive nature of rejuvenation. Successful rejuvenation is mental, physical, and spiritual. It begins within yourself and reaches to the highest planes of the cosmos. Once activated, it generates other powerful resources, including a more positive self-image, raised intellectual capacities (particularly memory and reasoning), and better physical health.

Rule 7. Master a variety of rejuvenation strategies. Through practice and experience, you will discover the procedures that work best for you. Incorporate into your plan strategies that target a variety of rejuvenation resources. Think of your rejuvenation efforts as a personal investment. They will give you a sense of control over your life. Keep in mind that some rejuvenation strategies will bring immediate results whereas others will require weeks, months, or even longer before their full effects are realized.

Rule 8. Relate your rejuvenation efforts to other personal goals. Rejuvenation procedures can significantly enhance other life pursuits, including academic and career success. The spin-off effects of rejuvenation can enrich your total life.

Rule 9. Be flexible. Open your mind to new ideas and new ways of enriching your life. Learn something new each and every day.

Rule 10. Embrace change. Whether to resist or embrace change is one of life's most important choices. Successful rejuvenation requires change—there can be no growth without change.

Rule 11. Develop a positive style of life. Believe in yourself and your power to succeed. Take good care of your mind and body. Exercise, eat right, and don't smoke. Avoid all negative entanglements that could thwart your growth. Keep in mind that unsinkable optimism and a fighting spirit are always rejuvenating.

They promote good health and increase longevity. Negative emotions—hostility, anger, resentment, worry, and anxiety—lower your defenses and make you more susceptible to disease.

Rule 12. Increase your awareness of your natural environment. Awareness spawns attunement. By increasing your awareness of your natural surroundings, you enhance your mental, physical, and spiritual well-being.

Rule 13. Enjoy life's simple pleasures. Having lunch with friends, playing afternoon cards, attending a favorite sports event, taking a moonlit walk, sharing fond memories with family or friends around a fireplace, watching a movie, playing a musical instrument, working out in the gym, curling up with an interesting book, hiking in the forest, riding horseback, or cruising down the river—all are rejuvenating, invigorating, and health enhancing.

Rule 14. Develop a healthy sense of humor. Humor is the Holy Grail of rejuvenation. It is intrinsically revitalizing and age defying. Every strategy presented in this book is enhanced by a robust sense of humor.

The list of fourteen rather than a conventional sum as embedded in our culture—the top 10, leading 25, best 100—rejects the notion that sets of principles, goals, guidelines, and so forth must be shaped or rounded out to conveniently fit a preconceived numerical format. This book does not hesitate to discard traditional constrictions, practices, and beliefs. For instance, the proposition that the crown of youth must eventually be lost, or that a long, youthful, quality life is available only to a privileged few is steadfastly rejected. We now know enough about the mind and body to alter the rigid programming that sets growth limits and energizes the aging process. We can revitalize weak neural connections, and when necessary, forge totally new ones. We can extinguish self-defeating attitudes, and create entirely new growth possibilities. We can be activists who reject the negative cultural stereotypes that fuel aging. We can learn exciting new ways of arresting aging and reversing its effects on the mind and body.

Even when the shadow of death eventually falls across our paths, the crown of youth prevails. Always, there is light behind the shadow. The bright peaks of all our past growth are instantly reclaimed at the moment of our transition to the other side. We are at once transformed by the renewal of all our accumulated life experiences. Fortunately, all the transforming power of our future transition is available to us in the here and now. Staying young and living a longer, more productive life are, at last, practical options for everyone.

Summary

Rejuvenation potentials are meant to be realized. By cultivating them, you can whet your appetite for exuberant living and enjoy life's grandeur to its fullest. Through the strategies presented in this book, you can discover exciting new ways of living younger, longer, and better. You can, at last, turn your back on aging with complete success.

In the chapters that follow, we will explore a wide range of elements, concepts, and strategies directly related to rejuvenation and longevity. We will introduce a total of forty-five strategies specifically designed to facilitate rejuvenation. Many of the strategies were developed in the college laboratory setting; whereas others are based on field studies, anecdotal accounts, and college classroom projects—all in an effort to discover new ways of living a younger, longer, and richer life. We will present strategies that defy aging by protecting and fortifying the self's innermost energy system. We will explore the mental and physical dimensions of rejuvenation, along with the higher cosmic sources of rejuvenating power. We will examine new ways of actively decelerating aging and, in some instances, literally reversing its effects. We will conclude by offering a seven-day plan designed to initiate an upward growth spiral that counteracts aging and promotes continuous renewal of the mind, body, and spirit. Always, our emphasis is on workable strategies that facilitate not only rejuvenation and longevity, but quality of life as well.

Because of the wide-ranging differences among individual preferences and characteristics, an optimal set of rejuvenation strategies appropriate for everyone has not yet been forthcoming. Only through exploring a variety of options, and occasionally modifying them to meet our personal and situational needs, can we find the approach that works best for us individually.

CHAPTER 2

Stress and Rejuvenation

Stress is an inevitable part of everyday life. None of us is immune to it. We each respond to it in different ways, depending on its nature and the coping resources available to us. Our personal empowerment and the success of our rejuvenation efforts depend largely on our effectiveness in managing stress.

Stress exists in two major forms—*positive* and *negative*. Positive stress is constructive energy that is potentially empowering both mentally and physically. It is a state of *attentive arousal* that inspires and motivates us to overcome obstacles and achieve goals. We generate positive stress when we set positive goals or commit ourselves to a worthy endeavor. It can emerge spontaneously when we encounter new opportunities for growth or face challenging situations that demand our best. It adds excitement to our lives, and it prods us to act constructively. It promotes effective problem solving and stimulates creativity. It saves us from boredom, and prevents atrophy. On the job, it prevents burnout and increases efficiency. It helps with mental alertness and clear thinking.

Positive stress helps us stay younger and live longer. At a physical level, it enlivens and rejuvenates biological functions. It is especially critical to the circulatory system and vital organs. It can help remove blockages and repair biological potholes. It helps the 40,000 miles of blood vessels in the body to nourish and rejuvenate the brain, heart, and other body organs which, without nourishment, would rapidly age and eventually die.

In contrast to positive stress, negative stress is corrosive energy that asserts a wear-and-tear effect on both the mind and body. It unleashes stress hormones in the blood; and it depresses the body's immune system. Even a mild degree of negative stress can, over time, slowly deplete our coping resources by weakening our mental and physical defenses. It can be subtle like a slowly gathering storm in the distance, or it can strike recklessly with the furor of a tornado spreading its dangerous debris. It accelerates the aging process, and in its most sinister form, it can lead to serious illness and even death.

We set the stage for negative stress by nurturing such feelings as inferiority, guilt, and worthlessness; harboring irrational beliefs; setting unrealistic expectations for ourselves; and giving in to an attitude of helplessness and despair. Other common sources of negative stress are excessive dependency, inflexibility, loss of hope and meaning, thwarted or unfulfilled strivings, separation from significant others, and a host of catastrophic life situations.

Negative stress tends to be cumulative in nature. At excessive levels, it exhausts our growth resources, impairs our efficiency, and predisposes us to failure, all of which can generate a vicious cycle of even more negative stress. If unattended, the accumulation of negative stress can eventually exceed our tolerance to cope with it—the result is a severe depletion of our adjustment resources and a breakdown of our coping mechanisms. In its most sinister form, negative stress can totally disarm the mind and body.

As negative stress increases, rejuvenating energies typically decrease. The result is an acceleration of aging along with a deterioration of the body's defenses against disease. Under excessive long-term stress, the body's immune system is eventually compromised, and we become even more susceptible to illness. If sufficiently severe and long-term, negative stress can be fatal. The gradual wear-and-tear effect on the body's organs and systems can result in failure of critical functions and finally, death. Effective stress management is, consequently, crucial not only to rejuvenation, but to life itself.

Fortunately, negative stress can be managed and its consequences controlled or extinguished altogether. Effectively managing negative stress is, in fact, one of the most powerful rejuvenation and health tools known. Our total personal empowerment is, to a great extent, dependent on our mastery of effective stress management strategies. We will later discuss several detailed procedures for managing negative stress.

Effective stress management is enhanced by certain underlying characteristics of the self. As a general rule, those self-characteristics which promote our personal growth likewise increase our ability to manage stress effectively. Here are a few examples.

- **Internal Locus of Control.** Recognize your inner ability to control your life and the forces that influence it. Studies of centenarians consistently revealed a sense of personal control over their lives. A strong inner locus of control spontaneously increases our stress coping skills.

- **Self-awareness.** Become aware of your strengths as well as your weaknesses. Your ability to use your strengths to compensate for your weaknesses is crucial in managing stress as well as achieving other important personal goals.

- **Self-insight.** Find time to reflect on your life and the meaning of your existence. You are much more effective in managing negative stress when you are focused and in touch with your innermost self.

- **Positive self-image.** Develop a positive view of yourself and an unwavering belief in your destiny for greatness. How others see you is not as important as how you see yourself. Recognize your imperfections as growth potentials. Think of problems as growth challenges. Have faith in yourself and the power within.

- **Balance.** Become attuned and balanced, both within yourself and with the cosmos. Balance is one of your best safeguards against negative stress.

- **Openness to Change.** Without change, there can be no growth. Openness to change increases your ability to create change and take command of your life.

- **Initiative and Motivation.** Know what you want for yourself. Don't hesitate to reach beyond yourself. Find ways of achieving your personal goals while making the world a better place for others.

- **Knowledge.** Knowledge is power. Increase your repertoire of problem solving and adjustment skills. Knowledge facilitates growth and adaptation.

The most effective stress-management approach emphasizes prevention over treatment. Although we can never completely escape negative stress, we can equip ourselves to thwart its invasion and repel its enfeebling effects. Rather than becoming overwhelmed by stress, we become stronger by exercising our inner coping and defense capacities. Effective stress management automatically activates our inner growth potentials and unleashes our dormant growth resources.

As we mature, effective stress management becomes even more important. We must fine-tune old strategies while acquiring new ones specific to our changing needs. The world changes and so must we. What worked in the past does not always work in the present. Among our major challenges is the discovery of new, advanced ways of satisfying personal needs, adapting to change, resolving conflicts, and solving problems. Meeting those challenges depends largely on our capacity to manage negative stress. Following are a few examples of negative stress situations and related stress management goals.

- **Our need to achieve is counterpoised by the fear of failure.** The fear of failure can overpower our drive to achieve important life goals. As a result, we withdraw in frustration and defeat. Effective stress management counteracts the fear of failure with positive expectations of success.

- **The search for meaning is opposed by the fear of self-discovery.** The need to know one's true self is often opposed by fear of discovering unacceptable impulses and strivings. Effective stress management recognizes and accepts imperfections as normal. Truth and fear fly to heaven on the same wing.

- **Goals are poorly formulated and efforts to achieve them are unfocused.** Our goals can be so ambiguous that they are unrealizable. Effective stress management identifies specific goals and formulates a decisive plan of action to achieve them.

- **Growth blockages are characteristically energized by negative stress.** All too often, we become victims of barriers that arrest our progress toward personal fulfillment. Effective stress management identifies the sources of blocked growth and musters the resources required to overcome them.

- **Excessive feelings of inadequacy and insecurity, along with low self-esteem, overpower the struggle for significance.** Negative feelings and perceptions are among the major sources of overwhelming stress. Effective stress management extinguishes negative elements and replaces them with feelings of personal worth and well-being.

These are only a few of the many stress conditions that, in the long haul, can accelerate aging. In the discussion that follows, we will explore several stress management strategies and their relevance to rejuvenation. Like all the forty-five strategies presented in this book, they are organized in logical steps to facilitate easy self-implementation. With practice, you will find each strategy increasing easy to use. Eventually, the steps become so automatic that the procedure flows almost effortlessly.

Strategy 1

Toe-Lift Technique

Simple physical relaxation is one of the most highly effective procedures for reducing negative stress. When combined with appropriate imagery and affirmation, physical relaxation can effectively unleash an abundance of rejuvenating energy. The Toe-lift Technique is specifically designed to (1) induce a deeply relaxed state, (2) extinguish negative stress, and (3) saturate the body's multiple systems and organs with rejuvenating energy. Here is the procedure which requires approximately 30 minutes.

Step 1. Preliminaries. In a comfortable, quiet setting, settle back and clear your mind of all active thought. Slow your breathing, and let all you cares gently roll away, like boulders rolling down a hill and into the sea.

Step 2. Toe Lift. Slowly raise your toes, and hold them in the raised position. If you are wearing shoes, press your toes gently against the top of your shoes. Hold the position as you sense tension building in your muscles, first in your feet and lower legs, then into your thighs, and finally throughout your body. Continue to hold the toe-lift position until the tension reaches its peak, typically within a minute or two.

Step 3. Relaxation. With the tension now at its peak, very slowly relax your toes, and allow them to finally reach their original position. With your toes now at rest, let the relaxation erase all tension by spreading gently upward, first into your ankles and lower legs, then slowly rising to infuse your total body. Take plenty of time for your body to become totally relaxed, from your feet to your forehead.

Step 4. Rejuvenating Mist. With your body now in a state of deep relaxation, envision a mist of bright, rejuvenating energy gathering around your feet and gently rising to envelop your total body. Sense your body absorbing rejuvenation from the tips of your toes to the top of your head.

Step 5. Glow of Youth. Breathe in the mist of bright rejuvenating energy, taking it deep into your lungs. Hold your breath for a moment, and allow the bright energies of youth to spread throughout your body, saturating joints, fibers, tendons, organs, and systems with radiant rejuvenating energy. Sense youthful vitality permeating every cell of your body. Envision your body enveloped in the glow of youth.

Step 6. Targeting Rejuvenation. Select specific physical signs of aging and mentally bathe each one with bright anti-aging energy. Envision rejuvenation as concentrated laser-like beams gently erasing the physical signs of aging and energizing your body's every function.

Step 7. Affirmation. As you remain deeply relaxed, affirm: *I am free of negative stress and fully infused with positive energy. Rejuvenation is now flowing throughout my total body.*

Step 8. Toe-Lift Cue. Conclude with the following rejuvenation cue: *I am empowered to eliminate negative stress and replace it with rejuvenation at any moment by simply raising my toes and affirming: I am relaxed and totally infused with the positive energies of youth.*

With practice, the Toe-lift Technique becomes increasing effective in managing stress and stimulating rejuvenation as well as building a positive state of personal well-being. The Toe-lift Cue (Step 8) can be used almost anywhere and under almost any condition to infuse the mind and body with positive energy. Wide ranging age groups have successfully used the cue for a variety of purposes. College students who practiced the procedure have used the cue to reduce test anxiety and improve performance, especially on tests requiring problem-solving and recall of large amounts of factual data. Along another line, an accountant, after practicing the full procedure, used the Toe-lift Cue to master his fear of driving across bridges with complete success.

Strategy 2

Control Center Strategy

Another highly effective stress management and rejuvenation procedure is the Control Center Strategy. This strategy recognizes the brain as the control center for the body with power to banish stress and induce rejuvenation. It focuses directly upon the brain and specific neurological responses that trigger negative stress reactions. The procedure does not, however, require special knowledge of the brain's complex structure and functions.

While the procedure recognizes the critical role of the brain as the body's control center, its primary emphasis is on the power of the mind to intervene into the brain's existing functions and to generate new ones. By simply relaxing the physical body and deliberately introducing certain imagery and new thought processes, we can shape brain activity and focus it on reducing negative stress, slowing the aging process, and reversing the biological effects of aging. Here is the procedure:

Step 1. Relaxation. Find a quiet, comfortable place, settle back, and focus your attention briefly on your breathing. Take in a few deep breaths, holding each breath for a few moments before slowly exhaling. Think of yourself as breathing in positive energy and exhaling negative energy.

With your eyes closed, develop a relaxed, rhythmic breathing pattern as you become more and more relaxed. Affirm: *I am calm, relaxed, and at complete peace with myself and the universe.*

Step 2. Brain Imagery. Center your thoughts on the dark, interior region of your brain. Envision your conscious presence in the brain as a light form illuminating the innermost regions and pathways of your brain.

Step 3. Brain Rejuvenation. Probe your brain's darkest central regions as you emit light from your conscious presence there. Slowly expel the darkness until your brain is aglow with bright energy. Allow the light of your presence to fully permeate your brain—energizing, rejuvenating, and revitalizing its activities. Your brain is now radiating bright, powerful energy.

Step 4. Inner Rejuvenation. From your control position at the brain's central region, use imagery to disperse positive energy in bright light form, first into your solar plexus region and from there, throughout your total body, driving away all the dark residue of negative stress until you are fully infused with light and positive energy. Bathe each physical organ with the light of health and rejuvenation. Take plenty of time to energize every physical organ and system with vitality and healing energy. Give stress-damaged and dysfunctional organs permission to heal and function normally.

Step 5. Outer Rejuvenation. While maintaining your control position in the brain, expand the energy emanating from your solar plexus until your physical body is enveloped fully in a powerful, expansive field of bright, rejuvenating energy. Give all outward manifestations of aging permission to slowly dissolve.

Step 6. Balance and Harmony. Envision your brain, solar plexus, and surrounding energy field interacting and working together in total harmony, all under the direction of your conscious mind.

Step 7. Rejuvenation Cue. As you envision yourself enveloped in bright energy, bring your fingers to your temples as a gesture to signify the infusion of positive, rejuvenating energy throughout your total being. Affirm in your own words your power to instantly reduce stress and activate rejuvenation at any time by simply closing your eyes and touching your temples as you envision yourself enveloped in powerful, bright energy.

After practicing this procedure a few times, you can effectively apply the Rejuvenation Cue (Step 7) as often as needed.

Strategy 3

Progressive Imagery Formula

Mental imagery is a critical component of almost all stress-management strategies. With practice, it can be used not only to induce relaxation but to activate rejuvenation as well.

The power of imagery to influence body tissue is based on the simple concept of "mind over matter." It embraces the premise that "whatever you envision, you can achieve." Aside from rejuvenation, a wide range of personal goals are responsive to imagery. Examples are breaking unwanted habits, overcoming fears, acquiring complex mental and physical skills, accelerating healing, fortifying the immune system, and achieving financial and career success.

The Progressive Imagery Formula is designed specifically to build basic imagery skills and apply them toward stress management and rejuvenation. The Formula introduces Regression Through Imagery (Step 9) to reach a state of youthful prime in which all signs of aging are erased. The procedure requires a small tangible item for object viewing and a full-length mirror for self viewing. Here is the procedure.

Step 1. Object Viewing. Select a small tangible item such as a piece of jewelry, flower, or art object, and take a few moments to view it. Focus your thoughts only on the item as you note its specific characteristics, such as size, color, structure, and so forth. Note the feelings that accompany the viewing process.

Step 2. Mental Imagery. Close your eyes and envision the selected object. Allow adequate time for a detailed picture to form clearly in your mind. Once the object becomes visible, note again the feelings that accompany your image. Note particularly the serenity and relaxation that usually emerge during the imagery process.

Step 3. Object Review. Again, view the object. Compare the object with the image you formed of it. Note the similarities and differences between the object and related image.

Step 4. Imagery Practice. Repeat the above steps until the viewed object is highly similar to the detailed image you formed of it. With each imagery exercise, note the serenity and relaxation accompanying the process.

Step 5. Self-Viewing. Having practiced your viewing and imagery skills, view yourself while standing before a full-length mirror, noting your specific physical features. Study your eyes, facial features, body proportion, and other distinguishing characteristics, to include any signs of aging.

Step 6. Self-Imagery. With your eyes closed, form a mental picture of your body as seen in the mirror. Note again your distinguishing characteristics. Sense the tranquillity and relaxation that accompany the imagery process.

Step 7. Self-Review. Again, view yourself in the mirror and compare the view with the image you previously formed of yourself.

Step 8. Self-Imagery Practice. Repeat the self-viewing and imagery process until the mental image is strongly similar to the reflection of yourself in the mirror.

Step 9. Regression Through Imagery. Settle back into a comfortable position, and with your eyes closed, envision yourself once again standing before a full-length mirror. Study as before your eyes, face, and body. Target any signs of aging and mentally erase them from your image. Envision all signs of aging as slowly vanishing until you are at your youthful prime. Note the colorful glow of youth enveloping your body. Slowly breathe in the radiant glow, and sense rejuvenating energy permeating your total being, from the inside out. Allow plenty of time for the signs of aging to vanish.

Step 10. Concluding Affirmation. Conclude the procedure with relevant affirmations such as the following: *I am filled with youthful vitality. Rejuvenation is unleashed to flow throughout my body. Mentally, physically, and spiritually, I am renewed, revitalized, and empowered.*

After a few practice runs using the full procedure, you will probably find that you can eliminate Steps 1 through 8 and go directly to Step 9 where your imagery skills are used as a regression vehicle to unleash rejuvenating energy. It is important to always conclude the procedures with appropriate affirmations.

Strategy 4

Fingertip Engagement Procedure

As we have already seen, a simple physical gesture can become a powerful tool for managing stress and stimulating rejuvenation. The Fingertip Engagement Procedure incorporates fingertip-to-fingertip touch into a step-by-step procedure designed to achieve three important goals, (1) reducing stress, (2) inducing a state of mental and physical harmony, and (3) activating rejuvenation.

Step 1. Body Scan. Settle back, take in a few deep breaths, and develop a slow, rhythmic breathing pattern. Close your eyes and mentally scan your body slowly from your head downward, pausing at tight, tense areas and releasing the tension. Let your total body become increasingly loose and limp.

Step 2. Energy Infusion. Turn the palms of your hands upward, and sense positive energy slowly gathering in the center of your palms. Let the accumulation of energy in your palms slowly radiate to energize both hands. You may sense warm, tingling sensations as the enrage builds in your hands.

Step 3. Fingertip Engagement. Slowly bring your fingertips together, one pair at a time beginning with the thumbs and progressing to the little fingers. Let each progressive engagement of the fingers represent a word in the five-word affirmation, "I am now fully empowered," with the thumbs signifying "I," the index fingers signifying "am," and so forth. Notice the sense of peace and harmony accompanying the gesture. Once all your fingers are engaged, mentally re-affirm: "I am now fully empowered." (Note: At this point, you can introduce other positive affirmations appropriate to your rejuvenation goals or current life situation.)

Step 4. Self-Empowerment Cue. Affirm in your own words your power at any time to reduce stress, generate balance, and activate rejuvenation by simply bringing your fingertips together as a gesture of full empowerment. Whenever difficult situations arise, you can use the self-empowerment cue to quickly release a powerful surge of positive energy.

Aside from its effectiveness in managing stress and promoting rejuvenation, this procedure is especially useful in combating phobias which, like stress, accelerate aging through their wear-and-tear effects on the mind and body. When practiced repeatedly, and with positive affirmations that target the phobia, such as, "I am empowered to face this fear and defeat it," the procedure reduces the fear and eventually extinguishes it altogether. The aging effects of persistent, uncontrolled fear are consequently eradicated.

Strategy 5

Inner Balance and Attunement Strategy

This strategy, while recognizing the asymmetrical make-up of the brain, emphasizes biological and mental balance as a critical component of stress management and rejuvenation. It focuses on the interaction between the mind and body, and the supreme power of the mind to induce a state of attunement and balance. Here is the procedure.

Step 1. Body Imagery. In a quiet, comfortable place, settle back and with your hands resting, palm sides upward, form a mental picture of your physical body at rest.

Step 2. Left Hand–Right Hand Imagery. Focus your full attention on your hands. Envision your left hand as representing the left side of your body, and your right hand as representing the right side of your body.

Step 3. Sensory Focusing. Lift your hands slightly, and notice the various sensations in each hand. Especially notice the tingling in your palms which represents energy frequency patterns. Compare the sensations in your left and right hands. Notice the similarities and differences, particularly in the weight of your hands and the energy frequency patterns registered in your palms.

Step 4. Praying Hands. Bring your hands together in a praying hands position. Sense the merging of energies, especially at your fingertips.

Step 5. Balance and Attunement. Allow the merging of energies in your hands to continue until you sense a full balance and attunement of frequency patterns. Once your hands reach a state of equilibrium, typically within a few seconds, separate them, and with each hand again turned palm side upward, let balance and attunement gently spread into your arms and then throughout your total body.

Step 6. Concluding Affirmation. Relax your hands and affirm: *The energies of my being are now fully attuned and balanced. The organs and systems of my body are at total harmony with each other. Mentally, physically, and spiritually, I am infused with the power of positive, rejuvenating energy.*

You can activate whenever needed the empowering potential of this procedure by simply bringing your hands together in a praying hands position as you affirm in your own words the procedure's balancing, attuning, and rejuvenating effects.

Strategy 6

Hand-Clasp Strategy

This procedure is similar in some ways to the Inner Balance and Attunement Strategy, particularly in its balancing effects. It is, however, a more assertive procedure in that it deliberately induces a state of physical tension in order to generate mental and physical balance. Here is the procedure which can be administered from almost any position.

Step 1. Left Hand Exercise. Form a tight fist with your left hand and hold it for a few moments as the tension builds in your hand and lower arm. Now slowly relax your hand, letting the muscles in your hand and arm become loose and limp.

Step 2. Right Hand Exercise. Repeat Step 1 using your right hand.

Step 3. Hand Clasp. Bring your hands together and clasp them tightly. Hold the tight clasp for a few moments as the tension builds and spreads upward into your arms and shoulders.

Step 4. Clasp Disengagement. Relax your hands, and allow them to come to rest in your lap or to your sides.

Step 5. Progressive Relaxation. Allow the relaxation in your hands to spread slowly upward into your arms, shoulders, chest, and finally, throughout your total body. Let every muscle, fiber, joint, and tendon of your body become deeply relaxed.

Step 6. Harmony and Balance. As you remain in a state of deep relaxation, close your eyes and note your sense of harmony and balance. Tell yourself that you are at complete peace with yourself and the universe.

Step 7. Rejuvenation. With your eyes remaining closed, envision rejuvenation as bright energy accompanying the relaxation process, revitalizing every fiber of your being with luminous energy. In your own words, affirm the harmonious, rejuvenating effects of the procedure.

Step 8. Postprocedure Cue. To reactivate the effects of this procedure at any time, simply repeat the Hand-clasp exercise (Steps 3 and 4) and follow it with affirmations of relaxation and rejuvenation.

Although the Hand-clasp Strategy and the Inner-attunement Strategy are similar, they are offered here as options, partly because of their separate appeal to different populations. Men and women college students along with older adult men who practiced both procedures typically preferred the Hand-clasp Strategy. Older adult women, on the other hand, preferred the Inner-attunement Strategy. Many of our subjects, however, believed they increased the rejuvenating effects of each strategy by using both.

Summary

This chapter presents numerous strategies for managing stress and alleviating its wear and tear effects on the mind and body. The two major forms of stress (positive and negative) are explored, and the personal characteristics associated with effective stress management are identified. The chapter presents several procedures designed to manage stress and promote rejuvenation. Practice with a variety of procedures is recommended in order to find the most workable approach. Each strategy is flexible and can be modified as needed to meet personal preferences and needs.

Chapter 3

Hypnosis and Rejuvenation

Hypnosis is an altered state of awareness in which our subconscious faculties and resources become increasingly receptive to our conscious probes. Hypnosis can range from a mild, relaxed state of increased receptiveness to a profound trance state in which consciousness is dramatically altered. At its deepest level, sometimes called the somnambulant state, memories buried deep in the subconscious can often be retrieved and critical subconscious resources activated.

In some instances, dormant potentials have been known to emerge full-blown during the deep trance state, a phenomenon known as hypnoproduction. Examples are fluency in a new language, advanced knowledge of a new discipline, and mastery of a new artistic or musical skill. One of my hypnosis subjects, a prelaw student who had just begun a course in French, spoke the language fluently while under hypnosis. Although he was unsuccessful in instantly transferring that advanced skill to the waking state, he used self-hypnosis to accelerate his mastery of the language. Along another line, a psychology student with no

history of psychic gifts discovered that she could accurately pre-
dict future events, some with important international significance, while in the trance state. Similar to the prelaw student's
experience, her remarkable ability, while not immediately apparent in the waking state, became increasing evident through her
practice of self-hypnosis.

In recent years, the therapeutic relevance of hypnosis has
become increasingly recognized among mental health professionals. The strategy is particularly effective in the treatment of
various anxiety and adjustment disorders. Other common applications are managing weight, breaking unwanted habits such as
smoking and nail-biting, reducing pain, managing weight,
building resistance to illness, and even accelerating healing.
There is an emerging body of evidence to suggest that hypnosis
can improve memory, increase motivation, stimulate creativity,
and even accelerate the rate of learning. As previously noted, the
technique can trigger precognition, as well as other important
psychic functions such as clairvoyance and telepathy. Given
these wide-ranging applications, it should come as no great surprise that hypnosis has important rejuvenation potential.

Hypnosis as a rejuvenation strategy is important in several
ways. First, it can set the stage for implementing a wide range of
age-management strategies. Examples are procedures that target
the underlying dynamics of aging as well as the external signs of
aging. Hypnosis is also important to rejuvenation because of its
capacity to energize inefficient biological systems, including
malfunctioning or weak organs. Furthermore, hypnosis can
influence brain activities in ways that directly alter the neural
and biochemical functions associated with aging. When appropriately applied, hypnosis as an age-defying strategy can slow the
aging process and literally reverse the visible signs of aging.

For rejuvenation as well as many other self-empowerment
applications, self-hypnosis is preferred over hypnosis administered by a trained professional. Given only limited practice using

appropriate procedures, almost everyone can master effective self-induction and trance-management skills.

(In a sense, all hypnosis can be seen as self-hypnosis. The model hypnotist, like the model therapist, exists within each individual. Without the cooperation of the inner hypnotist, the trance state will not occur.)

In self-hypnosis, the trance state is self-induced and self-managed. When used with certain precautions, and within appropriate guidelines, self-hypnosis is a safe and profoundly empowering procedure. Needless to say, it should not be used while driving a car, operating machinery, or in any work or recreational situation requiring vigilance or involving danger. The setting should be comfortable and free of distractions. Many subjects prefer soft background music or faint noise, such as distant street sounds, a waterfall, brook, or falling rain. Many subjects prefer the peaceful sounds of the open meadow for both relaxation and self-hypnosis.

The use of self-hypnosis as a rejuvenation tool is based on five important concepts:

- A vast reservoir of dormant yet powerful rejuvenating resources exists in the subconscious.

- Self-hypnosis can access that reservoir and draw healthful, rejuvenating energy from it.

- Self-hypnosis can literally alter the biological and psychological components of aging. Our so-called autonomic systems as well as subconscious processes are directly responsive to hypnotic intervention.

- Self-hypnosis can not only activate important rejuvenating interactions between the mind and body, it can introduce totally new anti-aging mechanisms.

- Self-hypnosis can empower us to overcome barriers that hinder our rejuvenation efforts.

Our conscious powers represent only a small fraction of our total potentials. Like the distant reaches of space, the subconscious mind is a vast region of exciting possibilities awaiting our probes. It consists not only of our past experiences not presently available to conscious awareness, it is also an intricate maze of potentially empowering mechanisms. Some of our subconscious mechanisms are only marginally active, whereas others are totally dormant. Through self-hypnosis, we can uncover that vast store of possibilities and use them to achieve our highest personal goals, including rejuvenation, while dramatically increasing the richness of our lives. Fortunately, the subconscious with its wealth of resources is always a willing partner in our rejuvenation efforts.

Despite conventional assumptions that aging is largely an uncontrolled physiological phenomenon which is determined largely by genetics, new emerging perspectives recognize the complex mental, spiritual, and physical interactions underlying aging as well as our capacity to deliberately influence them. Through self-hypnosis, we can eliminate subconscious age accelerants and introduce new age-defying interactions. We can uproot the aging influences of negative self-perceptions and replace them with positive self-awareness. We can identify the corrosive effects of aging on the mind and body, and replace them with youthful vitality. We can introduce totally new mechanisms that arrest aging, revive worn organs and stressed systems, and reverse the negative processes that energize aging. The result is a longer, richer, and healthier life.

Numerous self-induction and trance management strategies have been developed in recent years, and they are, as a general rule, easily mastered. The most effective strategies recognize the master hypnotist existing within each of us. Through self-hypnosis, we can awaken that inner specialist which, once activated, becomes a reliable and cooperative guide for our personal empowerment through the trace experience. A major spin-off reward of self-hypnosis is a deeper awareness and appreciation of the innermost self as a powerful life force with endless potential for growth.

The use of self-hypnosis, whether for rejuvenation or other goals, requires a safe, quiet, and comfortable setting. Approximately one hour should be allowed for the typical session during which there must be no distractions. Whether you are seated or reclining, your legs should remain uncrossed so as not to cut off circulation, with your hands resting comfortably to the sides of your body or on your thighs. The goals of hypnosis are usually formulated prior to the induction of the trance state. Through practice, inducing the trance state becomes more rapid and the effects of hypnosis more pronounced. Keep in mind that you can exit hypnosis at any time by simply giving yourself permission to end the trance state. A gradual exit, usually by slowly counting from one to five, is recommended over a rapid exit, which can leave any on-going interaction between the conscious and subconscious either incomplete or unresolved. If you decide deliberately not to end the trance state, you will eventually exit spontaneously or else you will drift into restful sleep. Self-hypnosis can, in fact, be used as an excellent sleep-induction technique.

Among the critical factors affecting the success of self-hypnosis as a rejuvenation strategy are a recognition of your inner rejuvenation potentials and a willingness to use them. In the following discussion, we will examine several trance induction options, each specifically designed to activate rejuvenation within the self system. For each strategy, the effectiveness of the trance state is enhanced by first, giving yourself permission at the start to enter hypnosis and use the experience to alter aging, and second, as the trance ensues, reassuring yourself that you are in full control for the duration of the experience.

Rejuvenation procedures using hypnosis typical include posthypnotic cues which can be used at any time following the application of the full procedure. Appropriate posthypnotic cues are important because they can be used to instantly activate the empowering effects of hypnosis. They can effectively strengthen the hypnotic suggestions while giving substance to the expected rejuvenation results. Even when nothing more than a slight gesture, the cue can awaken a myriad of subconscious potentials. The cue, with its accompanying affirmations, is usually more effective if presented just before ending the trance state.

Strategy 7

Hypnotic Rejuvenation Through Hand Levitation

Although numerous trance induction strategies are available to the self-hypnotist, a strategy particularly appropriate for rejuvenation is the hand levitation procedure. This strategy establishes a clear link between the mind and body, which is a critical component of age management and rejuvenation. Beyond its capacity to link the mind and body in a potentially empowering interaction, the strategy establishes a highly responsive mental and physical state in which a variety of rejuvenation procedures can be introduced. Here is the strategy.

Step 1. Preliminaries. Find a comfortable, quiet place and set aside approximately one hour for the session during which there must be no distraction.

Step 2. Cognitive Relaxation. Settle back into a comfortable seated or reclining position with your hands resting lightly on your thighs. Take in a few deep breaths, exhaling slowly, and clear your mind of all active thought. Develop a comfortable, rhythmic breathing pattern. Beginning at your forehead, mentally scan your body downward, pausing at areas of tension and allowing them to relax. Let relaxation soak deep inside your body from your forehead to the tips of your toes.

Step 3. Mental Imagery. Let relaxation go even deeper by envisioning a peaceful, relaxing scene. Examples are a peaceful sunset, perhaps with buildings or trees silhouetted against a golden sky; a white sail, drifting gently in the breeze; or a billowy cloud moving slowly across an azure sky. (Note: When imagery of movement is introduced at this stage, a left to right direction is usually more effective.)

Step 4. Hand Levitation. With your body now deeply relaxed, affirm in your own words your intent to enter hypnosis and use the experience to activate rejuvenation. Remind yourself that you can exit hypnosis at any time by simply deciding to end the trance state. Then center your full attention on your hands resting on your thighs. Without moving your hands, notice each specific sensation—the weight of your hands, the pressure at your fingertips, the texture of your clothing, the warmth or moistness in your palms, and the coolness at the top of your hands. Next focus your full attention on your right hand, again noticing each sensation in that hand as it continues to rest on your thigh. As your focus stays centered on your right hand, notice the sensation of lightness, as if a slight pressure under your hand were pushing it upward ever so gently, or as if a balloon were tied loosely around your wrist, gently pulling your hand upward. As your hand begins to rise, give yourself permission to enter the trance state as soon as your hand touches your forehead. Remind yourself that you will remain in full control for the duration of the trance experience. Allow plenty of time for your hand to levitate until it touches your forehead. Then close your eyes and let your hand slowly return to your thigh.

Step 5. Trance Deepening. To deepen the trance state, slowly count backward from ten, interspersing suggestions of going deeper along the way.

Step 6. Trance Testing. Test the trance state as follows. (1) Select a certain body area, such as a finger, and induce

a particular sensation, such as numbness, warmth, or coolness. Then remove the sensation and allow the area to
return to normal. (2) Select two body reference points,
such as the ankle and knee, and induce a particular sensation as before in the body region between the two points.
Then remove the sensation and allow the region to return
to normal. If you are successful in inducing the selected
sensations, go to the next step. If you are unsuccessful in
inducing the sensations, return to Step 5 to further deepen
the trance state.

Step 7. Rejuvenation. As the trance state continues, present your rejuvenation goals using positive affirmations
and, where possible, related images as follows for (a) cosmetic rejuvenation, (b) corrective rejuvenation, and (c)
rejuvenation of mental functions:

a. Cosmetic Rejuvenation. Cosmetic procedures are used
to erase the visible signs of aging. Envision yourself standing before a full-length mirror, with your body enveloped
in a colorful glow of rejuvenating energy (select any pastel
shade you prefer). Affirm: *I am enveloped in a radiant glow
of youth and vitality. As I breathe in the powerful glow,
youthful vitality is unleashed to flow throughout my total
body. All the visible signs of aging are vanishing. I am filled
and overflowing with rejuvenating energy.*

b. Corrective Rejuvenation. These procedures are used
to energize biological organs and systems with rejuvenation. As a particular organ or system is visualized, bright
energy emanating from the body's solar plexus is directed
to infuse the designated target. The organ or system is then
envisioned as brightly illuminated with new energy. Affirm:
*My total body, inside and out, is infused with the energies of
youth. Day by day, the dull mechanisms of aging will surren-
der to the bright instruments of youth.*

c. Rejuvenation of Mental Functions. To rejuvenate
mental functions, envision the brain glowing with bright

vitality. Think of your conscious awareness as bright energy, and focus your full awareness on various interior regions of the brain. Mentally stimulate the brain, replacing dull regions with the brightness of your conscious presence. Linger long enough to fully illuminate the brain. Target specific functions, such as memory, problem solving, vocabulary, language, creativity, and so forth, and mentally stimulate them. Affirm: *The abundant powers of my mind are constantly at my command. They are in a state of complete readiness, poised to respond as needed.*

Step 8. Hypnotic Affirmations. In your own words, affirm your power to use the enormous resources existing in your subconscious. An affirmation example: *The rejuvenation mechanisms of my subconscious are now at their functional peak. All the rejuvenating resources of my subconscious are now unleashed to permeate my total being with the energies of health and youth.*

Step 9. Posthypnotic Cue. Here are four affirmations, any one of which can be presented at this step and used following hypnosis as a posthypnotic cue to reactivate the procedure's rejuvenating effects. Select the affirmation which has the greatest appeal to you personally. (1) *By simply touching my forehead as I envision the glow of rejuvenating energy enveloping my physical body, I can instantly infuse my total being with positive rejuvenating energy.* (2) *I am empowered to instantly extinguish the aging process and replace it with rejuvenation by simply envisioning myself at my youthful prime.* (3) *I am empowered to instantly arrest aging and stimulate rejuvenation at any time by simply taking in a deep breath and exhaling slowly.* (4) *I am empowered to arrest aging and activate the rejuvenation process throughout my body by simply bringing my palms together and rubbing them gently against each other.*

Step 10. Conclusion. Simple intent to return to the normal waking state is usually sufficient to end the trance experience. The empowering effects of the trance are, however, strengthened by a slow exit, typically by counting from one to five, with suggestions of increased alertness.

Strategy 8

Object Illumination Procedure

Another self-hypnosis strategy designed specifically to tap the subconscious reservoir of rejuvenating energy is the Object Illumination Procedure. This procedure uses a small shiny object as a focal point upon which full attention is centered to induce the trance state while simultaneously unleashing rejuvenation. Like other induction approaches, this procedure requires a quiet, safe, comfortable setting.

Step 1. Preliminaries. For the seated position, situate a small shiny object, such as a thumbtack or adhesive star, on a wall so as to facilitate comfortable gazing. For the prone position, situate the object on the ceiling, again so as to facilitate comfortable gazing. Give yourself permission to experience hypnosis, and affirm your ability to end the trance state at any time through intent alone.

Step 2. Eye Fixation. Settle back and from your seated or prone position, give yourself permission to enter hypnosis and use it to achieve your rejuvenation goals. Then focus your gaze on the object, without tilting your head backward. Let your mind become free of all active thought as you gaze only at the object. If your eyes tire, close them for a few moments and then continue gazing at the object.

Step 3. Focal Shift. Following a brief period of gazing, slowly expand your peripheral vision, first taking in the immediate area surrounding the object, then progressively expanding your peripheral vision to its limits. Once your peripheral vision reaches its limit, let your eyes fall slightly out of focus. You will immediately notice a white, milky glow surrounding the object and expanding throughout your visual field. Allow this effect to continue for several moments, then slowly close your eyes.

Step 4. Trance Induction. With your eyes now closed, notice deep relaxation spreading throughout your body. Affirm: *As I count slowly backward from ten, each number will take me deeper and deeper into hypnosis. I will come out of hypnosis at any moment by simply deciding to end the trance state. I will remain in full control throughout the trance experience.* Count slowly backward, interspersing suggestions of going deeper and becoming more fully relaxed. Upon the count of one, affirm: *I am now in hypnosis and responsive to each of my suggestions.*

Step 5. Rejuvenation Release. Envision a bright, radiant mist around your feet and slowly rising. Allow sufficient time for the mist to rise and fully envelop your body, then affirm: *I am now totally infused with the energies of youth and health. All organs and systems of my body are now renewed with healthful vigor.* At this point, you can supplement this step with additional affirmations that target specific health needs or rejuvenation goals.

Step 6. Posthypnotic Cue. Before ending the trance state, affirm: *I am empowered to reactivate the rejuvenating effects of this procedure at any time by simply envisioning a bright, energizing mist slowly rising to fully envelop my body.*

Step 7. Conclusion. To end the trance state, slowly count from one to five, while suggesting alertness and full wakefulness. On the count of five, affirm: *I am now fully alert and at my peak of rejuvenation.*

Strategy 9

Finger-Spread Procedure

Yet another excellent hypnotic strategy for unleashing rejuvenation is the Finger-spread Procedure. This procedure, which was developed in our laboratories at Athens State University, requires spreading the fingers of either hand and then slowly relaxing them to induce the trance state. Trance induction through the Finger-spread Procedure is similar to the hand levitation technique in that it combines mind control and motor activity to establish a positive mind-body connection, with mental functions assuming dominance over physiology. Such a connection not only facilitates rejuvenation, it generates a deeply relaxed and mentally focused state conducive to a host of other self-empowerment goals, including pain management and weight control. Here is the procedure.

Step 1. Preliminaries. Find a quiet place, and assume a comfortable position with your hands resting either at your sides or on your thighs. Give yourself permission to enter hypnosis, and affirm your ability to exit the trance state at any time by simply deciding to do so.

Step 2. Trance Induction. Spread the fingers of either hand, and hold the spread position as your hand begins to tire. Continue to hold the spread position as the tension in your hand spreads into your arm. Allow the tension in your hand to reach its peak, then begin to very slowly relax your hand. Give yourself permission to enter hypnosis as your hand becomes increasingly relaxed. Let the two processes—relaxation and hypnosis—emerge slowly and concurrently. Think of the two processes as related but separate, with the mind assuming dominance over the body. Take plenty of time for the two functions to occur simultaneously. Suggestions of going deeper and deeper and becoming more and more relaxed facilitate the emerging trance state. If you sense the two processes progressing at different rates, adjust the relaxation state so that the two processes occur together.

For instance, if the relaxation in your hand seems to progress faster than the trance process, hold the existing relaxation state until the trance state reaches the same approximate level. On the other hand, if the trance advances too rapidly, accelerate relaxation until the two process reach similar levels. These adjustments will require practice, but once mastered, they will ensure an effective trance state.

Step 3 (Optional). Trance Deepening Strategies. Although the Finger-spread Procedure typically produces a trance state sufficient for rejuvenation, deepening strategies are sometimes required to reach the optimal level of hypnosis. Examples of effective deepening strategies include (1) reverse counting, typically from ten, with interspersed suggestions of relaxation and drowsiness; (2) a wide range of mental images, such as a pebble tossed into a cerulean pool and slowly sinking to the bottom, or slowly moving objects such as a sail or billowy cloud drifting in the breeze; and (3) manipulation of sensory processes, by inducing and then removing or relocating isolated sensations, such as tingling, numbness, warmth, or coolness. A common deepening technique is to induce and then remove numbness in a finger, followed by suggestions of depth and drowsiness. Typically, you will sense when an appropriate trance level has been reached.

Step 4. Rejuvenation. With mental dominance over physiology established through the trance induction procedure, targeting rejuvenation to various physical destinations becomes a natural mental process. Mental imagery of desired rejuvenation outcomes, such as the elimination of certain physical signs of aging or the revitalization of specific biological organs and systems, is combined with positive affirmations to activate a powerful rejuvenation interaction. The combination of two dynamic age-defying faculties—visualization and verbal power—within the context of mental dominance over physiology is usually sufficient to awaken dormant rejuvenation potentials.

Subconscious sources of rejuvenation—including the anti-aging mechanisms that revitalize the body and restore youthful vitality—are particularly responsive to this strategy. At this stage of the procedure, a warm, gentle flow of revitalizing energy typically accompanies the rejuvenation interaction between mind and body. It is important to allow adequate time for the rejuvenation process to run its course.

Step 5. Posthypnotic Cue. The Finger-spread Procedure can be used as an excellent posthypnotic gesture for activating the rejuvenation effects of this procedure. To establish the cue, simply affirm: *I am empowered to activate rejuvenation at any moment by simply spreading the fingers of my hand* (the same hand as used in the induction procedure) *and then slowly relaxing them.*

Step 6. Conclusion. To end the trance state, slowly count from one to five, while suggesting alertness and wakefulness.

With practice using any of the above trance induction options, many subjects acquire the remarkable skill of rapidly entering the trance state through sheer intent alone as well as initiating at will the mind-body interaction. Simply settling back and, with eyes closed, affirming: *I will now enter hypnosis,* is the simplest and possibly most advanced form of trance induction known.

Although self-hypnosis, once mastered, is an invaluable source of anti-aging and rejuvenating power, its capacity to alter the aging process is only one of its many applications. Of particular relevance to rejuvenation is its use in breaking the smoking habit and managing weight. Both smoking and excessive weight not only pose serious health risks, they also accelerate aging. Fortunately, each of the induction strategies discussed above can be easily adapted to achieve these important goals.

When applied to smoking, hypnosis can build determination and self-confidence in one's ability to master the smoking habit while generating a powerful new image of oneself as a "successful nonsmoker." The procedure first introduces powerful affirmations of determination and success during the light to moderate trance state. It then interjects relevant imagery and appropriate posthypnotic suggestions to assure total success. Here is an example:

> *I am determined to break the smoking habit. I have more than enough power to succeed in achieving this goal. Beginning now, I am free of this habit. If I am offered a cigarette, I will simply say, "No, I am a nonsmoker." If I find myself reaching for a cigarette, I will say, "No." If I find myself thinking about smoking, I will say, "No." The word "No" is one of the most powerful words in the English language. I will use it whenever needed to totally break the cigarette habit once and for all.*
>
> *I can now envision a blank screen upon which appears the word, "No." This word represents my power over this habit. Simply envisioning the blank screen with the word "No" at any time will remind me that I am now a nonsmoker. I will be instantly empowered with total success.*

Envisioning the blank screen and the word "No" can be used whenever needed as a posthypnotic cue to build determination and ensure complete success in breaking the smoking habit.

As a weight management strategy, which requires appropriate medical supervision, self-hypnosis again uses a combination of affirmations, imagery, and posthypnotic cues. Here is an example.

> *My goal is to weight exactly* (state the amount). *I am determined to achieve this goal. I will eat only the foods that are good for me. I will eat slowly, relishing every bite. I will thoroughly enjoy eating, but only in the amount required to reach my goal. As I succeed, I will become invigorated and rejuvenated. I can now envision myself standing before a full-length mirror, weighing exactly* (state your goal). *This is the true "me" which I have held prisoner behind excessive weight.* (Here, be careful not to state "my excessive weight" which denotes ownership). *At any time, I can empower myself with determination and success by simply*

clasping my hands and envisioning myself weighing exactly (state amount). *I now give myself permission to succeed in this effort. I will achieve my goal. I am destined for success.*

For most personal empowerment goals, including weight management, habit control, and rejuvenation, self-hypnosis and related posthypnotic cues typically require frequent practice, particularly in the early stages of the empowerment plan.

Rejuvenation Through Hypnotic Regression

Rejuvenation through hypnotic regression is yet another application of self-hypnosis in mastering the aging process. Hypnotic regression is based on the concept that, as an evolving conscious entity, we are at any moment the totality of our past experiences. A variation of that concept is the view that the subconscious is a vast repository of all experience not presently known to consciousness, including our development in all our past lives. Even our existence before our first incarnation as well as our life between lives is chronicled within the archives of the subconscious. Those hidden experiences, many of which are charged with rejuvenation energies, challenge us to explore them and unleash their capacity to empower our lives. The act of participating in this discovery effort can be equally as empowering as the end-discovery itself. Uncovering and activating the extensive resources of the subconscious—to include the accumulated experiences of our distant past—is one of our major and most rewarding lifetime tasks.

Because many of our past experiences, having been stored in the subconscious, are outside of conscious awareness, strategies that probe the subconscious are required to uncover them. Hypnosis (along with such strategies as dream analysis and free association) can part the curtain to reveal crucial events of the past, often in a dramatic and highly detailed reenactment.

Regression through hypnosis consists of two major forms (1) current lifetime regression—typically called age regression—and

(2) past-life regression. Age regression explores experiences which occurred during our present incarnation, from our earliest prenatal development in the womb to the present. Past-life regression, on the other hand, delves into our most distant past to explore three important dimensions (1) our existence before our first incarnation, commonly called *preincarnate existence;* (2) our past incarnations; and (3) our existence in the discarnate realm between our past lives. In all its forms, hypnotic regression enables us to re-experience past events as though they are present realities.

Among the concerns regarding regression as a rejuvenation strategy is the possibility of uncovering painful, threatening past experiences buried in the subconscious. The best safeguard against such a possibility is the formulation of clear, positive objectives prior to induction of the trance state. Positive goal statements tend to generate positive results. When presented early in the procedure, they function as gate keepers to hold at bay all irrelevant or potentially damaging experiences. The stated intent of tapping your dormant rejuvenating potentials is usually sufficient to focus the trance experience and bring forth only positive results.

Although certain applications of hypnosis require a skilled professional with specialized training in hypnosis as a clinical procedure, many of the goals of hypnosis, including certain regression applications, can be achieve through self-hypnosis. As we previously noted, all hypnosis can be seen as self-hypnosis. Since the best potential hypnotist exists within the self, it would follow that self-hypnosis, when used with appropriate safeguards, can be effectively applied toward tapping subconscious rejuvenation resources, which are linked to our past.

Hypnotic regression is relevant to our rejuvenation efforts in a variety of ways:

- Simply experiencing the peaks of our past growth is spontaneously rejuvenating. When we regress to those peaks and linger in the regressed state, we become mentally and physically renewed. That process is enriched by step-by-step procedures that highlight relevant past events.

- The regression experience can uncover influences that contribute to aging. Past-life enlightenment can dissolve growth blockages and resolve conflicts that could inhibit our rejuvenation efforts.

- Hypnotic regression often reveals cosmic or spiritual guides from the past who are poised to assist us in our rejuvenation efforts.

- A more complete understanding of our past through hypnotic regression can enrich our lives with new power and a deeper understanding of our life's purpose and destiny.

Each of us is one person with many past lives. When we add to them the abundance of our experiences between our past lives along with our existence before our first incarnation, we are overwhelmed by the wondrous possibilities of probing our past. Once we are equipped with knowledge from our personal past, we can take greater command of the present and more effectively shape our future growth.

Strategy 10

Rejuvenation Through Age Regression

The goal of Rejuvenation Through Age Regression is twofold: first, to create a peak infusion of rejuvenation for persons who are beyond their peaks of youth and vitality (typically the late teens or early twenties); and second, to stimulate a continuous flow of rejuvenation within the self. Here is the procedure.

Step 1. Trance Induction. Induce the trance state using any of the trance induction procedures previously discussed.

Step 2. Age Regression. Once you achieve the trance state, envision a staircase with the top of the staircase representing the present and the base of the staircase representing your past developmental peak of youth and vitality. Envision yourself slowly descending the staircase, step-by-step, with each step taking you further back into your past. Envision each step slowly erasing the physical signs of aging. Upon reaching the base of the staircase, you are at your developmental peak of youth and vitality.

Step 3. Anti-Aging Infusion. As you linger at the base of the staircase, envision a full-length mirror with yourself standing before it. View yourself at your youthful prime, infused with healthful energies and bathed in the glow of radiant youth. Breathe in slowly and deeply to fully absorb the energies of youth.

Step 4. Peak Infusion and Balance. Let the infusion process continue until it reaches its peak. Now fully imbued with the energies of youth, generate a state of complete mental, physical, and spiritual balance by briefly touching your temples with your fingertips as you affirm in your own words the balancing effects of the gesture.

Step 5. The Return. To return to the present, slowly climb the staircase, step-by-step, as you remain totally energized and enveloped in the glow of youth. Note the spring in your step as you ascend the staircase.

Step 6. Rejuvenation Cue. Upon reaching the top of the staircase, affirm in your own words your power to activate on command the rejuvenating and balancing effects of the trance experience by simply closing your eyes at any time and briefly touching your temples with your fingertips.

Step 7. Conclusion. To end the trance state, count slowly from one to five while interjecting suggestions of being awake and fully alert. Upon the count of five, open your eyes and briefly reflect on the rejuvenating effects of the experience.

As noted in Step 6, you can activate at any time the procedure's rejuvenating and balancing effects by simply closing your eyes and briefly touching your temples. The long-term effectiveness of this cue is heightened by periodically applying the full procedure.

Strategy 11

Rejuvenation Through Past-Life Regression

This procedure is based on the premise that each one of us is the totality of all our past experiences, including our past incarnations. Rather than distant incarnations existing separate from our present life, our past lives are seen as integral components of our presence existence. Existing primarily in the subconscious, past-life experiences, while remaining largely unknown to most of us, are an ever-present influence on our behavior. That influence, while potentially empowering, is too often uncontrolled and underused.

A major role of each incarnation is the continuous integration of past incarnations into our present development and evolution. Our knowledge of the past helps us to meet the demands and challenges of the present. Rejuvenation Through Past-life Regression is specially structured to access dormant rejuvenation resources which, while linked to our past lives, are presently available to us through our probes of the subconscious. The procedure recognizes the amazing capacity of the subconscious to select potentially rejuvenating past-life experiences and convey them during the trance state to conscious awareness. The result is a fully activated interaction between our conscious rejuvenation needs and the essential subconscious resources required to fulfill them. Here is the procedure.

Step 1. Goal Statement. In your own words, state your rejuvenation goals. Examples include erasing the physical signs of aging, arresting the aging process, and revitalizing internal organs and biological systems.

Step 2. Trance Induction. Induce the hypnotic state using any of the trance induction procedures previously discussed.

Step 3. Cognitive Relaxation. To deepen the trance state, let yourself become more fully relaxed by mentally scanning your body from your head downward. You can facilitate this process by envisioning relaxation as a luminous mist gently settling over your total body. Envision every muscle, joint, and fiber of your body absorbing the radiant mist.

Step 4. Cognitive Passivity. With your body now aglow with relaxation, focus your full attention on your breathing. Let each breath take you slowly back in time until you experience a state of "nothingness" in which your mind is a blank screen. At this state, initiate no active thought. Let yourself experience only the blank passivity of your mind. •

Step 5. Past-Life Imagery. After a few moments in the passive mental state, remind yourself of your rejuvenation goals, and let related images of your past-life spontaneously emerge. Remind yourself that the subconscious part of yourself is empowered to select the appropriate past-life images. Think of these images as rejuvenating energy forms with power to renew and revitalize your mind and body.

Step 6. Past-Life Rejuvenation. Let the emerging series of past-life images become established in your conscious awareness. Once the subconscious past-life experiences are firmly registered in consciousness, sense the energy interaction between the images and your physical body. Note the rejuvenating, energizing sensations throughout your body. Focus your attention on specific body regions and allow rejuvenating energy to fully permeate them. Affirm your power to defy aging and master it fully. Envision the glow of youth enveloping your full body.

Step 7. The Return. To end the regression experience, focus your full attention again on your breathing. Let each breath take you a step forward in time until you are again in the present moment. It is important to take plenty of time for your return to the present, since a rapid, abrupt disengagement of the past can negate the procedure's rejuvenation effects.

Step 8. Posthypnotic Suggestion. Once your return to the present is complete, tell yourself that you can call forth at will specific regression images that will instantly initiate a powerful anti-aging interaction within your mind and body. At this step, you can designate a specific cue, such as lifting a toe while visualizing a luminous mist enveloping your body, to activate the procedure's rejuvenating effects.

Step 9. Conclusion. To end the trance state, count slowly from one to five, while interspersing suggestions of becoming alert and fully awake.

Subjects who use this procedure usually experience a wide range of past-life images with immediate rejuvenating effects. Colorful images involving important past-life achievements and physical prowess are not unusual. A fifty-one-year old stockbroker, with serious inferiority feelings, experienced past-life images of her role as a strong warrior who victoriously led men into battle. The experience empowered her to take command of her life. She became more energetic, and she developed new social and recreational interests. Even her physical posture improved, a reflection of the renewal effects of the procedure.

Along another line, a mechanical engineer, age forty-eight, with serious health problems, experienced during regression a series of past-life images depicting his role of tribal medicine man. Subsequent regressions resulted in a progressive improvement in his health status, which he attributed to a combination of past-life enlightenment and the rejuvenating effects of regression on his physical body.

$$\boxed{\textit{Strategy 12}}$$

Discarnate State Regression

Discarnate State Regression differs from other regression procedures in that it focuses on either our existence before our first incarnation (pre-incarnate existence) or else the discarnate intervals between our past lives rather that on our past incarnations. The purpose of this procedure is twofold (1) to retrieve essential rejuvenation resources generated during our past discarnate existence, and (2) to tap the vast reservoir of subconscious knowledge related to longevity and rejuvenation, much of which also seems to have been acquired during our past discarnate existence. Like Rejuvenation Through Past-life Regression, this procedure recognizes our capacity during the trance state to spontaneously select potentially rejuvenating discarnate resources and to use them to empower our lives in the present.

This procedure is based on the concept that our growth evolved, not only during our past lives, but also in the discarnate realm, often in the company of higher guides, advanced teachers, and growth specialists. In those intervals of our development, we acquired a vast amount of knowledge, to include concepts related to longevity and rejuvenation. Like many of our past-life experiences, much of that knowledge may have been lost to conscious awareness. Nevertheless, it continues to exist in the vast regions of our subconscious where it, fortunately, can become available to us through Discarnate State Regression. Through this procedure, we can tap into our past discarnate existence and retrieve the valuable knowledge stored there.

This procedure, unlike conventional past-life regression, makes no direct effort to uncover past-life identities or incarnations. Although relevant past incarnation experiences will sometimes surface spontaneously during the procedure, they do not typically take center stage, but rather provide the backdrop for discarnate resource materials to emerge.

Discarnate State Regression, which views the discarnate state as a higher dimension of existence, is based on our present capacity to experience that higher reality. As we will later see in this book, we can directly experience the discarnate dimension as it presently exists through a variety of strategies, but to understand that dimension as we personally experienced it in the past can reconnect us to its powerful influence on our total existence. When we reconnect to that dimension as we knew it, we invariably experience a revival of its rejuvenating capacity.

Aside from its direct rejuvenating effects, this procedure reveals the magnificence of the discarnate realm, with its wondrous opportunities for our continued evolvement. When death eventually leans against the door, our transition to the discarnate dimension becomes a magnificent gateway to new growth and renewal. But aside from providing an open door for our continued development, our passage into that realm instantly transforms and restores us to our past peaks of youth and achievement. The effects of aging, injury, and disease are instantly erased by our transition to the other side. Therefore, it should come as no great surprise that our brief excursions into that dimension are both healthful and rejuvenating.

The preferred induction strategy for this procedure is the upward gaze technique, a very rapid but easily mastered trance induction strategy. This technique is often accompanied by a sense of "raised consciousness," in which awareness of higher dimensions of reality frequently emerges spontaneously. Here is the procedure.

Step 1. Goal Statement. In your own words, state your intent to enter the discarnate dimension of your past development. Clearly formulate your objectives, with emphasis on the healthful, rejuvenating possibilities of the procedure.

Step 2. Trance Induction Through the Upward Gaze. Settle back into a relaxed position with your hands resting comfortably on your thighs. Focus for a few moments on your breathing, and develop a slow, rhythmic breathing pattern. With your eyes open, gaze upward but without tilting your head backward. While continuing to gaze upward, slowly close your eyes, and once your eyes are closed, let them return to normal. Sense the relaxation around your eyes gently spreading over your total body as you drift deeper and deeper into the trance state.

Step 3. Trance-Deepening Strategy. To further deepen the trance state to the desired level, center your attention on either hand as it rests on your thigh. Note the weight of your hand, along with sensations of warmth, coolness, tingling, texture of your clothing, and so forth. Now selectively focus your attention on your little finger. Note the sensation of numbness, first at the tip of your little finger, then spreading slowly along the outside of your hand, and finally over your full hand. Allow the numbness to remain for a few moments, and then give permission for the feeling to return to your hand. Move your little finger to signal that the feeling has returned. At this point, you can further deepen the trance by counting slowly backward from five as you interject suggestions of becoming drowsy and going deeper.

Step 4. Discarnate Regression. Having reached the desired trance level, focus your full attention again on your hands. Assign to each finger a particular interval between past lives, with the little finger of your right hand representing your most recent discarnate interval, and the little finger of your left hand representing a very distant interval. As you center your attention on each finger, beginning with your right little finger and moving progressively backward to your right thumb, and then from your left thumb and moving progressively backward to your left little finger, you will sense on which finger to arrest your focus. If your attention is not arrested on the first round of counting, repeat the rounds until your attention is finally arrested on a particular finger. Focus your full attention on the selected finger, and give yourself permission to regress to that discarnate interval. Allow awareness of that interval to fully emerge, typically within only a few seconds of focusing. Once awareness occurs, let yourself fully experience the interval as an active participant, not simply a casual observer. Provided you clearly formulated your goals in Step 1, the subconscious discarnate experiences relevant to those goals will typically emerge spontaneously. Let yourself fully absorb the rejuvenating energies of that discarnate interval and the conscious-subconscious interactions related to it. Take plenty of time for the process to run its course.

Step 5. The Return. Once the regression experience has run its course, let yourself return to the present by first shifting your attention back to the finger representing the selected discarnate interval. From that finger, move forward by focusing your attention on each finger until you reach the little finger of your right hand. Finally, move that finger as a signal that you have returned to the present.

Step 6. Posthypnotic Cue. In your own words, tell yourself that by focusing your full attention at any time on the finger selected for this regression experience, you can instantly activate the procedure's rejuvenating effects.

Step 7. Trance Exit and Conclusion. To end the trance experience, count slowly from one to five, pausing briefly after each count to suggest wakefulness and alertness. On the count of five, open your eyes and take a few moments to reflect on the experience.

A majority of our subjects using this procedure for the first time arrested their focus on the middle finger of the left hand (Step 4), which represented their eighth past-life interval. Interestingly, the number eight, according to numerology, signifies success and fulfillment. In subsequent sessions, they arrested their focus randomly among various fingers.

As a footnote, several of our subjects found that they could easily modify Step 4 of this procedure to deliberately regress to their earliest pre-incarnate state, thus uncovering important life experiences occurring before their first incarnation. To regress to that state, they simply continued the rounds of counting until they sensed having reached beyond their most distant between-life interval, whereupon their pre-incarnate experiences typically emerged in very bright and colorful imagery form.

As noted in Step 5, you can at any time instantly activate the rejuvenating, anti-aging effects of the procedure by simply focusing your attention on the finger selected to represent the regression experience.

Summary

The innermost part of our being, to include the deepest levels of our subconscious, is always responsive to the powerful hypnotist within. Through self-hypnosis, we can become increasingly empowered to master our own lives and the forces that influence us, including the aging process.

Simply experiencing the trance state can be enlivening and rejuvenating. But when we use self-hypnosis as a rejuvenation strategy, all the accumulated resources of our past and present can become readily available to us. By awakening our dormant inner potentials, self-hypnosis activates a powerful renewal process that enriches the quality of our lives—mentally, physically, and spiritually. By probing our past, to include our past lives and our past experiences in the discarnate realm, self-hypnosis spans our total existence to unleash abundant new growth energy and greater understanding of the magnificent cosmic nature of our lives. This powerful technique is one of the most important rejuvenation and growth options available to us today.

CHAPTER 4

Sleep and Rejuvenation

On average, we spend about a third of our life sleeping. As Shakespeare noted, "Our little life is rounded with a sleep!" To ignore this important part of our existence could seriously affect the quality of our lives and limit our achievement of important goals, including rejuvenation.

Sleep is a critical component of successful rejuvenation for several reasons:

- It generates an ideal biological and mental state with empowerment potential for everyone.

- Restful sleep is spontaneously rejuvenating. To quote Shakespeare again, it "knits up the raveled sleeve of care." Regular, healthful sleep (around eight hours daily) prevents the wear and tear that can shorten our lives.

- Like self-hypnosis, the sleep state is highly responsive to our deliberate intervention.

- Powerful rejuvenation mechanisms lie dormant in the subconscious. Sleep intervention techniques can effectively activate them.

- When appropriately managed, the drowsy state *immediately preceding* sleep can set the stage for successful rejuvenation *during* sleep.

- Dreams are the golden highway to rejuvenation. Through appropriate dream intervention, we can awaken the rejuvenation process and effectively channel rejuvenating energy to designated mental and physical goals.

- The awakening state immediately following restful sleep can be used to unleash new rejuvenating energies as well as to reinforce the rejuvenating effects of sleep.

Several strategies have been developed in our laboratories at Athens State University to maximize the rejuvenation potentials of sleep. Certain of these strategies are highly nonintrusive—they are designed primarily to promote restful sleep. They are typically used to enrich the spontaneous, anti-aging functions of sleep. Other strategies, however, are more intrusive—they are designed to profoundly alter the sleep experience. They often employ mechanisms that actively probe the subconscious and activate dormant rejuvenation potentials. They can include pre-sleep and dream intervention techniques that target specific subconscious anti-aging mechanisms. The most effective approach will include a combination of both intrusive and nonintrusive strategies.

During sleep, we are more highly receptive to the inner influence of the subconscious as well as certain higher plane influences of the cosmic realm. A potential spinoff benefit of sleep strategies is the discovery of personal cosmic guides. They are often rejuvenation specialists who intervene during sleep and especially during dreaming to guide our rejuvenation efforts. Although our best rejuvenation specialist probably resides within the deeper part of ourselves, higher cosmic specialists are important because they can put us in touch with that inner specialist. Furthermore, cosmic specialists themselves can be a source of totally new rejuvenating energy. In a later chapter, we will explore higher plane interactions and their relevance to rejuvenation.

Strategy 13

Sleep Enrichment Strategy

Everyone can benefit from the Sleep Enrichment Strategy, a nonintrusive procedure that promotes restful sleep while strengthening the normal rejuvenating role of sleep. It incorporates physical relaxation, mental imagery, and positive affirmations in a procedure that is implemented just prior to falling asleep. Aside from inducing restful sleep, the procedure protects sleep from inner disruptions, including the distressful invasion of anxiety. It is structured to energize the subconscious and awaken a variety of dormant anti-aging mechanisms. Although the procedure makes no effort to probe the deeper subconscious, it often generates insight and quality subconscious solutions. Notwithstanding these important benefits, rejuvenation remains the procedure's primary goal.

Step 1. Controlled Breathing/Body Scan. As you prepare to fall asleep, take in a few deep breaths and exhale slowly. Focus your full attention on your breathing while developing a rhythmic breathing pattern. As you continue to breathe slowly and rhythmically, mentally scan your physical body, beginning at your forehead and slowly progressing downward. Mentally bathe areas of tension with relaxation, as your body becomes progressively loose and limp.

Step 2. Mental Passivity. Briefly review the day's activities, including any important meetings, events, interactions, or other concerns, then allow them to gently fade away. Think of them as puffy clouds that slowly vanish,

leaving behind only the clear blue sky. This simple technique, which requires only a few seconds, clears the mind
and generates brainwave patterns that are conducive to
restful sleep.

Step 3. Visualization. Your mind now clear, visualize
yourself at your prime of life, with your body enveloped in
a radiant youthful glow. As you breathe slowly and rhythmically, imagine yourself soaking in the rejuvenating glow.
Let the glow of youth spread throughout your body,
slowly erasing the signs of aging and revitalizing your total
being. Sense the peace and tranquillity accompanying the
rejuvenating process.

Step 4. Affirmation. Silently affirm that as you sleep, each
breath will ensure a peaceful and continuous infusion of
youthful energy.

Step 5. Sleep. Let restful, rejuvenating sleep ensue.

You will find that, like most rejuvenation efforts, practice
increases the effectiveness of this procedure. But given even limited practice, most subjects drift easily into restful sleep at Step 5.
If sleep does not occur as expected, simple repeat the procedure,
going more slowly the second time around.

The research subjects who participated in our development of
the Sleep Enrichment Strategy frequently reported the appearance of a personal guide or higher plane cosmic specialist during
sleep. In one rather spectacular instance, an electrical engineer
reported the recurring visitation during sleep of a radiant guide
who imparted a luminous glow to envelop his body in a brilliant
aura of energy. The guide then gently massaged the surrounding glow to totally infuse and revitalize his body with abundant
new energy.

Another research subject, a thirty-eight-year-old fashion
designer, despondent over the recent loss of her mother,
reported several joyful visits during sleep by her mother, who

shared a variety of humorous happenings that occurred on the other side, one of which involved a slip of the tongue. As a result of the visitations, the designer successfully resolved her grief, and she began to more freely express her own sense of humor. As we noted earlier in this book, humor is the Holy Grail of rejuvenation.

| Strategy 14 |

Sleep Anti-Aging Strategy

This bold strategy is designed to manipulate sleep and redirect it in an effort to awaken dormant age-defying functions. It views sleep as a pliable resource, which can be shaped to achieve wide-ranging rejuvenation objectives. It plants images in the subconscious and uses them as rejuvenation tools. Dormant inner resources are awakened and directed toward specific objectives.

This procedure emphasizes both physical and mental renewal. In our laboratory trial runs, individuals of wide-ranging age differences reported a variety of positive effects. Mood state improved markedly for all participants. Memory as measured by the participant's ability to recall the content of passages presented to them verbally likewise improved. All participants reported the rejuvenating effects of the procedure on the physical body to some degree. Our studies found that, for best results, the three-step procedure should be used at least twice weekly.

Step 1. Presleep Conditioning. Prior to falling asleep, reflect on your immediate and long-term rejuvenation goals, both physical and mental. State them clearly in your mind, and think of them as not only goals but also future realities. Using imagery, assign to each goal a bright, crystalline form, with each luminous form representing a biological system or mental function to be revitalized and renewed. For instance, a cube can represent healthy cell reproduction, a pyramid can represent mental alertness, and a sphere can represent a strong immune system. Envision the forms as small enough to hold in the hand.

Step 2. Imagery. With your eyes closed, envision your subconscious mind as a clear pool of abundant rejuvenating energy. Picture yourself at the edge of the pool with the crystalline forms in your hands. Imagine yourself tossing the forms, one by one, into the pool. As each form sinks deeper and deeper, remind yourself that the fluid energy enveloping each form is saturating the mental or physical function it represents. Sense the flow of rejuvenating energy permeating your body. Continue to envision the clear pool with its crystalline forms until sleep ensues, typically within a few minutes.

Step 3. Postsleep Conditioning. Upon awakening, review your rejuvenation goals and affirm your power to achieve them. Envision again the clear pool with its crystalline forms. As you hold the image clearly in your mind, erect a triangle by first joining the tips of your thumbs to form its base and then joining the tips of your index fingers to form its top. Affirm that by simply forming the so-called Triangle of Power as you envision the pool with its forms, you can instantly activate at any time the flow of rejuvenating energy throughout your body.

The Sleep Anti-aging Strategy is a highly flexible rejuvenation procedure which can be easily revised to fit personal preferences. You can add more imagery and suggestions related not only to rejuvenation but other empowerment goals as well. A marine biologist, who was an avid swimmer, envisioned diving into the pool following casting the geometric forms into it (Step 2). For him, this added step dramatically increased the procedure's rejuvenating effects. Along another line, an art student tossed an irregularly shaped rock instead of a geometric form into the pool to stimulate creativity and improve the quality of his art works.

The Triangle of Power as a rejuvenation gesture can be used as often as needed to reinforce the effects of the full procedure. Because the gesture is relaxing as well as rejuvenating, it can also be used to effectively reduce stress and generate a powerful sense of personal well-being.

Strategy 15

Dream of Youth

Certain changes in dreams almost always accompany the use of rejuvenation strategies. On average, dreams become more frequent and are typically more vivid. They are usually more positive and rewarding. For older adults, they often involve regression to their youthful prime. In their dreams, women regain their beauty and men regain their youthful prowess. It would seem plausible that if rejuvenation stimulates certain changes in the dream state, then changes in the dream state could stimulate rejuvenation. The Dream of Youth strategy is based, in part at least, on that premise.

Imagery is the language of the subconscious. During the drowsy state immediately preceding sleep, the subconscious is especially responsive to imagery. As a presleep strategy, the Dream of Youth generates images that are then readily transferred to the subconscious. Once registered in the subconscious, imagery serves two major functions (1) it becomes the substance of the dream experience, and (2) it activates the dormant potentials related to the imagery. For instance, the image of yourself at your peak of youth, once received by the subconscious, generates the related dream experience and activates the rejuvenation resources required to achieve that image. Here is the procedure.

Step 1. Presleep. As you prepare to fall asleep, take in several deep breaths, exhaling slowly. Focus for a few moments only on your breathing.

Step 2. Finger Spread. Spread the fingers of either hand and hold the spread position until your hand begins to tire. As you slowly relax your hand, affirm in your own words your rejuvenation goals—both mental and physical. Continue to relax your hand until it is loose and limp. Sense the relaxation in your hand spreading into your arm and then throughout your body.

Step 3. Subconscious Interaction. As you remain drowsy and relaxed, address your subconscious as the innermost part of yourself and your partner in your rejuvenation efforts. Form clear images of yourself at your prime of youth, full of energy and glowing with health and vitality. Allow these images to sink deep within yourself. You will sense when they reach the deepest level of your subconscious.

Step 4. Affirmation. Affirm that as you sleep, your dreams will be a source of rejuvenation, insight, and power. More specifically, affirm the capacity of your subconscious to materialize your images of rejuvenation.

Step 5. Rejuvenating Sleep. Continue to envision your rejuvenation goals until sleep ensues.

This procedure, while designed specifically for rejuvenation-related goals, can be easily adapted to other personal empowerment objectives, to include career, social, and personal issues. In a remarkable example, a student used to procedure to find the love of her life. After she envisioned the "ideal mate" in Step 3, her subconscious accepted the image and returned it to her as a dream with only slight alterations. The dream continued until she eventually met the "man of her dreams." By her report, he matched exactly the person depicted in her dreams, down to a diagonal scar on his earlobe, the result of a childhood injury.

Strategy 16

Awakening Rejuvenation

Awakening from sleep, like falling asleep, is a transitional process in which the subconscious is especially receptive to conscious intervention. By capturing the few moments of somewhat semi-consciousness characterizing the natural awakening state, we can gain important access to a vast array of inner rejuvenation resources. Awakening Rejuvenation is designed to achieve that important goal.

This procedure requires either spontaneous awakening or gradual awakening, such as to soft music or other pleasing sounds. Abruptly awakening to a sudden alarm interrupts transitional awakening and inhibits the procedure's effectiveness. When sound recordings are used for awakening, it is important to select sounds that appeal to you personally. Many of our subjects made their own recordings, which included sounds of a New England meadow, the ocean, a rainstorm, busy city streets, and a train in the distance. Here is the procedure, during which your eyes remain closed for each step.

Step 1. Body Imagery. As you begin to spontaneously awaken from sleep, form an image of your physical body as it continues to rest comfortably.

Step 2. Facial Renewal. Imagine yourself with a pencil eraser in hand, gently erasing the visible signs of aging, such as lines around your eyes or mouth. To restore youthful muscle tone, visualize yourself placing a comfortable mask of youth over your face. Sense the firmness in the muscles as your face conforms to the mask.

Step 3. Full-Body Renewal. Envision yourself slipping into a form-fitting rejuvenation garment. Sense the gentle shaping of your body to the youthful proportions of the garment.

Step 4. Aura of Youth. Envision the mask and garment slowly fading, taking with them the signs of aging and leaving behind only the radiance of youth. Sense the glowing aura of youth enveloping your body.

Step 5. Inner Renewal. Envision the central region of your body radiating a youthful glow that saturates your total being, inside and out. Allow rejuvenating energy to infuse every organ and system of your body.

Step 6. Concluding Affirmation. Affirm: *Throughout this day, I will be at my peak of power and youthful vitality. The energies of youth will flow continuously throughout my total being.*

Like other sleep-related strategies, Awakening Rejuvenation is a flexible procedure that can be adapted as needed to meet highly specific rejuvenation goals as well as a wide range of health and fitness needs.

Summary

The sleep state offers an ideal condition for rejuvenation. Sleep is, by nature, renewing and revitalizing. By deliberately intervening into the sleep experience, we can direct it toward specific rejuvenation goals, thereby maximizing sleep's rejuvenating capacity. As a road to the subconscious, sleep gives us access to a wealth of subconscious resources, including rejuvenation. Both the presleep state and the awakening state offer further opportunity to maximize the rejuvenating capacity of sleep. An added benefit of sleep strategies is the discovery of higher plane cosmic guides who are rejuvenation specialists. By interacting with them, we can discover important new sources of rejuvenation and personal power.

CHAPTER 5

Rejuvenation and Higher Plane Interactions

We have probably learned more about the physical universe in the past decade than in the past century. Yet we have, at best, barely tinkered at its borders. It spreads magnificently before us, commanding our wonder and compelling us to probe its depths and boundaries. The more we explore the universe, the more we are amazed at its magnitude and splendor. Yet even more amazing is the real possibility that the physical universe as we know it is only one of many physical realities. In all probability, vast domains of physical realities, including other universes, exist beyond the borders of the physical universe as we currently conceive it.

Even more amazing than the existence of tangible reality, however vast it may be, is the existence of intangible reality, including many higher cosmic planes we could call spiritual. Like the physical universe, the nonphysical challenges our probes; and as with tangible reality, the more we probe the intangible, the more we are struck with awe at its magnitude and splendor. A better understanding of intangible higher planes, including the discarnate realm, is critical to our present existence, partly because it increases our understanding of ourselves and our place in the larger cosmic scheme.

Like the tangible and intangible dimensions of the cosmos, we are both physical and nonphysical. Our biological makeup, to include our genetic characteristics, provides only the basic raw materials for our development in this lifetime. As we interact with our physical environment, our attitudes, values, emotions, and cognitive skills emerge within the biological context of our being. But biology alone cannot explain our existence as a conscious, indestructible life force whose origin and destiny are cosmic, not biological.

To reach our highest destiny, we must transcend our biological boundaries and overcome our environmental limitations. Fortunately, we can expand our growth options by taking command of our biological resources. This can be objectively demonstrated through biofeedback procedures that literally monitor the power of the mind over biological processes. Blood pressure, body temperature, pulse rates, body chemistry, immune functions, and even brain wave patterns are all responsive to our deliberate intervention. Perhaps even more astounding, we can establish new neural connections and literally initiate new rejuvenating interactions within the brain.

Along another line, the power of the mind to influence external conditions independent of physical contact or intermediate instrumentation further reflects the wondrous power of the mind over physical reality. This phenomenon, typically called psychokinesis (Pk), suggests a near unlimited capacity of the mind to control matter. Examples include inducing motion in a stationary object, such as a pendulum, or mentally slowing an object already in motion. Given the human ability to influence inanimate matter at a spatial distance, it would follow that we could, with even greater ease, influence the biological body, to include repairing and even regenerating diseased body organs through sheer mind power. The concept of psychic or spiritual healing is based on that premise. (For further discussion of this topic, see my book *Psychic Empowerment for Health and Fitness.*)

Further reflecting the nonphysical nature of our being is our capacity to interact with higher spiritual realities. These interactions include but are not limited to (1) the peak experience in which we often experience a total oneness with the universe; (2) the near-death experience in which we temporarily experience the discarnate realm; (3) a wide range of miraculous events, to include unexplained healings; (4) the out-of-body experience that can include visitations to distant realities, including the other side; and (5) the many meaningful interactions with departed loved ones, angels, and ministering guides.

Our studies of life after death consistently showed that discarnates, upon their transition to the other side, not only retained their identity, personality, and conscious awareness; they also regained the peaks of all their past development, including the youthful prime of their immediate past life. The effects of aging, illness, and injury instantly vanished at their transition. Mental impairments and physical imperfections were replaced by radiant beauty. In the experimental situation using a variety of discarnate communication strategies, including the séance and channeling, as well as table tilting which is discussed in a later chapter, discarnates without a single exception described their transition to the other side as a transformation process that elevated them to a new level of either "wholeness" or "illumination." Confirming these findings are the numerous case studies of personal interactions with discarnate teachers and ministering guides. Perhaps even more important, discarnate interactions strongly suggest that the rejuvenation powers reflected in the transition to the other side are available to us now on this earth plane, and with equally powerful results. Through deliberately interacting with higher planes, we can access totally new and untapped sources of rejuvenation, enlightenment, and power.

Our surveys of subjects, all over the age of seventy-five, who appeared to retain many of the characteristics of their youth, almost always revealed a positive attitude about life after death. They typically did not fear death, but saw it simply as a door ajar, a new adventure, or an exciting gateway to a new level of growth. They often saw the "after-life" dimension as a "present-life" reality. Many of them experienced an ongoing interaction with a spirit guide or significant others on the other side. They often attributed both their excellent health and youthfulness to these interactions.

It is important to keep in mind that our spontaneous interactions with higher planes are always purposeful and potentially empowering. They can help us to understand ourselves, our origins, and our destiny. They affirm the existence of a spiritual reality and our intimate connection to it. They are a source of important knowledge, inspiration, comfort, and power. They affirm the eternal existence of our conscious identity. They teach us that we are active participants in a grand scheme of endless growth and discovery. They affirm that, when the physical body finally fails, the spirit not only survives, it thrives as well.

In view of the evidence that even casual interactions with discarnate realities are rejuvenating, it would seem plausible that structured strategies could be designed to tap the rich rejuvenating resources of higher planes, including the discarnate realm. Like hypnotic regression to the discarnate realm as previously discussed, our purposeful interactions with that dimension as it presently exists can lift awareness to a new level while renewing the mind, body, and spirit.

Several strategies for probing higher cosmic planes and accessing their resources have long been available to us. Typically interactive in nature, some of them were designed to communicate directly with the departed, whereas others were designed to interact with spiritual guides or teachers. Among the common examples are mediumistic communications, automatic writing, and the use of various tangible tools such as the pendulum and table (as used in table tilting). Although these strategies can yield important information, they are not typically structured to access specific growth resources. (We will later find, however, that table tilting can be applied as a rejuvenation procedure.)

In summary, rejuvenation through higher plane interactions is based on the following five premises:

- Higher planes, including the discarnate realm, are an infinite source of power and rejuvenating energy. (As noted in an earlier chapter, hypnotic regression to our past discarnate existence consistently reveals life in that dimension as inherently rejuvenating.)

- Higher planes offer an array of growth specialists—advanced teachers, ministering guides, angels, and a host of discarnate entities.

- Manifestations and interventions of higher plane origin, including the presence of personal guides and the visitation of angels, are always purposeful and empowering.

- The abundant resources of the higher planes are readily available to everyone. Certain planes are rich repositories of special resources. Even brief excursions into those planes can be inspiring, rejuvenating, and potentially healing to the mind, body, and spirit.

- Once mastered, procedures that tap higher plane sources of rejuvenation can be applied to achieve other important life goals, such as health and fitness, solutions to personal problems, spiritual insight, and resolution of grief, to list but a few.

The rejuvenation strategies that follow, while often expanding awareness and knowledge, are specifically structured to tap the rejuvenating resources of higher planes. As we explore our inner anti-aging potentials, it is important to keep in mind that the higher cosmic energies which constantly sustain the universe and our existence in it are readily available to us in the here and now. Higher plane strategies introduce us to some of the most powerful known sources of rejuvenation. They are designed to make higher plane realities accessible to anyone who is willing to explore them. As with other rejuvenation approaches, only through practice can we discover the higher plane procedures that work best for us individually.

Strategy 17

Cosmic Infusion Procedure

This procedure is designed to tap the highest cosmic source of rejuvenation energy. It views cosmic energy as white light which can be readily accessed and absorbed throughout the body to infuse it with rejuvenation and balance. Here is the procedure.

Step 1. Goal Statement. In a quiet, comfortable setting, affirm your goal of achieving a state of full cosmic infusion of rejuvenating energy—mentally, physically, and spiritually. State your rejuvenation objectives as specifically as possible. Examples include slowing the aging process, revitalizing the mind and body, activating inner anti-aging processes, erasing the physical signs of aging, strengthening and enhancing specific brain functions, and restoring mental and physical powers, to mention but a few of the possibilities.

Step 2. Relaxation. As you remain quiet and comfortable, settle back and take in several deep breaths, pausing briefly between breaths. Continue to focus on your breathing until you develop a comfortable, rhythmic breathing pattern. Think of each breath as "taking in" relaxation and "letting go" tension. Let your muscles become loose and limp as you release all physical tension, replacing it with deep relaxation.

Step 3. Energy Infusion. Turn your palms upward and think of your hands as your body's antennae to the cosmos. Envision the discarnate realm as a dimension of pure white light. Let bright beams of cosmic light enter your palms and then spread throughout your total body, balancing and energizing your total being. Sense the energy soaking deep into every fiber, muscle, and joint, infusing every vital organ and system with rejuvenation. (At this point, you may experience warm, tingling energy, first in your palms and then deep within your body.) Target rejuvenating energy to specific body areas. Allow plenty of time for the infusion event to reach its peak.

Step 4. Conclusion. Affirm your power to tap at will the resources of higher planes, and to use them to achieve your rejuvenation goals.

Although the effects of this procedure are often evident following a single practice session, with repeated practice the procedure becomes increasingly effective as an anti-aging strategy. The procedure, which is appropriate for any age group, can be practiced at any time and as often as preferred. Interestingly, college students using the procedure typically preferred a late afternoon hour for practice; whereas older adults typically preferred an early morning hour.

Strategy 18

Balance and Attunement Strategy

A critical key to rejuvenation is balance and attunement. All too often we are out of balance within ourselves and out of tune with the cosmos. When we are inwardly balanced mentally and physically, we are poised for growth. But when we reach beyond that inner state and become outwardly attuned to the cosmos, we have access to the highest sources of rejuvenating energy.

The Balance and Attunement Strategy is designed first, to produce a balanced and attuned state in which the mind, body, and spirit interact in complete harmony; and second, to tap outer cosmic sources for a powerful infusion of rejuvenating energy. It focuses on (1) the solar plexus as a physical energy center, (2) the brain as a mental energy center, and (3) the hands as a functional area for the accumulation and distribution of cosmic energy. The procedure is based on the following assumptions:

- The mind, body, and spirit are in a state of continuous interaction. Every individual is, at any point in time, the totality of that interaction. Each human function—whether mental, physical, or spiritual—interacts with every other function.

- The solar plexus is a critical region for physical interaction, the brain is a critical region for mental interaction, and the hands are critical regions for cosmic interaction.

- We function best when we are balanced and attuned—mentally, physically, and spiritually.

- If left unattended, our functions can become unbalanced and unattuned.

- When we are unbalanced and unattuned, we are out of harmony within ourselves and with the cosmos.

- When we are balanced and attuned, we are at harmony with ourselves and the cosmos. We can deliberately intervene to balance and attune each of our mental, physical, and spiritual functions.

- Balance and attunement are healthful and rejuvenating mentally, physically, and spiritually.

Here is the procedure.

Step 1. X Formation. While resting in a comfortable, relaxed position, cross your arms to form an X over your chest. As your arms remain crossed, think of your hands as antennae for your brain, with your right hand representing the brain's right hemisphere, and your left hand representing the brains left hemisphere. This gesture prepares your mind, body, and spirit for balance and attunement.

Step 2. Hand-Body Contact. As your arms remain crossed, simultaneously touch your left shoulder with your right hand and your right shoulder with your left hand. Hold the touch position for several moments as you sense the energy interaction between your hands and shoulders, and the emerging harmony deep within your solar plexus. Sense the inner balance between the right and left hemispheres of your brain as they function together in perfect accord.

Step 3. Praying Hands. Uncross your arms, and bring your hands together in a praying hands position. Note the powerful exchange of energy between your hands as you become increasingly attuned and balanced.

Step 4. Cosmic Infusion. Turn your palms upward, and envision radiant cosmic energy gathering in your palms. Sense the powerful infusion of energy, first in your palms, then in your solar plexus, and from there, radiating throughout your body. Note the sense of attunement accompanying the radiating energy.

Step 5. Energy Targeting. Mentally target rejuvenating energy to specific body regions. Let anti-aging energy melt away the effects of aging. Use your hands to distribute rejuvenation through physical touch. Use both imagery and touch to guide anti-aging rays of energy to designated targets—including any external sign of aging.

Step 6. Resolution. Again bring your hands together in a praying hands position. Affirm: *I am fully attuned and balanced mentally, physically, and spiritually.*

This strategy is especially useful in reversing the effects of premature aging associated with physical illness or long-term stress. Aside from its rejuvenating effects, subjects who practice the procedure often report significant improvements in mood state and increased effectiveness in coping with stress. College students who practiced the procedure immediately before examinations reported an increase in their ability to think clearly and remember important course material. When practiced regularly, the procedure resulted in dramatic improvements in grade-point averages for both men and women students.

Strategy 19

Cosmic Interaction Strategy

While attuning and balancing your energy system with higher cosmic energy sources are important to your rejuvenation efforts, the discovery of higher plane entities—particularly rejuvenation specialists—can further enhance your success in mastering the aging process.

Higher plane entities from the cosmic realm often enter our lives spontaneously, particularly at times of personal distress or danger. They can help us find solutions to difficult problems, overcome growth barriers, and resolve personal conflicts. They can intervene to comfort us in times illness, grief, and tragedy. They can prepare us for difficult situations, protect us from unseen danger, and guide us toward personal fulfillment. Many of our so-called "peak experiences" and "flashes of insight" appear to involve interactions with ministering guides. Given these manifestations, it should come as no surprise that cosmic rejuvenation specialists can help us open new growth channels and increase the inner flow of rejuvenating energy. Cosmic Interaction Strategy is a high intensity procedure designed specifically to achieve that goal.

Rejuvenation specialists are critical growth facilitators who guide and energize our growth, especially during the formative years of life. Many children come to know them as "imaginary" playmates or friends, and even assign them names. But as we mature, we tend to drift away from them, and over the years, the gap widens. This procedure narrows that gap by reintroducing us to them and establishing new interactions with them. Although the primary goal of the procedure is the direct transfer of rejuvenating energy of cosmic origin, other important benefits almost always come forth. Here is the procedure.

Step 1. Letting Go. Settle back and, with your eyes closed, clear your mind of all active thought. Then, as you remain relaxed, allow new thoughts and images to slowly flow in and out of your mind. Make no effort to arrest these thoughts and images as you experience the calming effects of simply "letting go." Allow this free-flowing process to continue until smooth tranquillity replaces the ragged edges of stress.

Step 2. Childhood Reverie. As you remain in a passive, relaxed state, allow images of your childhood to flow in and out of your mind. Let the images freely come and go until a particularly pleasant image of an early childhood event enters your mind. Focus on the event for a few moments, then give yourself permission to drift back in time to re-experience it exactly as it occurred. Allow plenty of time to become completely absorbed in the unfolding event. In that state of reverie, sense the wonder of your childhood and the freedom from all your accumulated cares.

Step 3. Cosmic Infusion. Now free of your adult baggage, let yourself sense anew the inner attunement and oneness with the cosmic source of your existence. As you linger in the reverie state, note your feelings of wondrous congruency with the cosmos. Sense the nurturing resources of the higher cosmos, and remind yourself that they are now available to you. Expand your awareness to include the presence of ministering guides and teachers along with caring angels and other spiritual helpers, some of whom will probably seem familiar to you. Take plenty of time to renew your awareness and appreciation of them. Remind yourself that they are your present helpers. You can invite them to guide your pursuit of rejuvenation as well as other important goals in your life. Sense the rejuvenating power of your interactions with them as the glow of youth envelops your body. Let the interaction and energizing process continue until your are fully infused with rejuvenating cosmic energy.

Step 4. Into the Present. The cosmic infusion process now complete, shift your attention to the present and your immediate surroundings. Remind yourself that the supreme cosmic forces that energized your existence from the beginning are constantly present to enrich your life with all the abundant resources of the cosmos.

Step 5. Conclusion. Affirm your ability to reactivate the effects of this procedure at any time by simply reflecting on the early childhood experience and opening your mind to the wondrous presence of higher plane entities.

Almost everyone who practices this procedure experiences a sense of wonderment at their rediscovery of "forgotten" higher plane acquaintances. A forty-year-old engineer, who rediscovered the angel who had been his childhood companion, remarked, "I was reunited with a wonderful friend from my past." An eighteen-year-old college student experienced a reunion with the spiritual guide who had comforted her as a child when her father died in an auto crash. She described the reunion as a peak experience she would never forget.

Strategy 20

Higher Plane Rejuvenation

The cosmic dimension consists of numerous higher planes, each with its own unique energies and empowerment potentials. From a spiritual perspective, physical reality as we know it is merely a tangible manifestation of an intangible life force. That force, rather than a parallel to physical reality, is the essence of reality and the sustaining force that energizes it. Without that force, energy and life in their multiple forms would cease to exist. Just as the essence of the physical body is its life-force counterpart, so is the essence of the universe. Coming to know that sustaining life force—both within ourselves and in the outer cosmos—is a major purpose of our existence on this planet. Ultimate growth can be defined as a complete oneness with that inner and outer life force.

Our laboratory studies, using various altered states—hypnosis, meditation, dreams, and the out-of-body experience—revealed the existence of numerous energy planes found throughout the cosmos. Each plane was found to have its own design, col-oration, and energy frequency as well as its unique function. Our studies further showed that we can access the resources of vari-ous cosmic planes and use them to enrich our lives. We found, for instance, that structured interactions with planes of yellow could significantly enhance memory and other intellectual func-tions as measured by standardized tests. Interactions with light-blue planes, on the other hand, were useful in generating a peaceful, tranquil state of mind. We found the light-blue plane to be a critical resource in the clinical treatment of anxiety and depressive disorders.

Our studies found that interactions with bright-green planes were particularly effective in promoting health and fitness. Per-formance in the gym setting markedly improved following the use of either hypnosis or structured out-of-body experiences as strategies for experiencing the green plane. Immediately fol-lowing their interactions with the green plane, our subjects invariably demonstrated a dramatic increase in stamina and endurance.

Based on our laboratory studies spanning a period of several years, we developed a procedure specifically tailored to access the green plane as a source of rejuvenating energy. Similar in some

ways to the Balance and Attunement Strategy previously discussed, this strategy, called Higher Plane Rejuvenation, specifically targets an expansive green plane which appears to be
situated near the bright center of the cosmos. The procedure
identifies the radiant core of the cosmos as a concentrated form
of life-force energy. The iridescent green plane, which is directly
energized by the cosmic core, transforms pure life-force energy
into a rejuvenating form that is responsive to human interaction.
By interacting with the green plane, we can revitalize and renew
the physical body. Following the procedure, a radiant, healthful
glow usually envelops the subject, an effect that can be quite
profound, even for the skeptic. Here is the procedure, which
requires about thirty minutes in a setting free of distractions.

Step 1. Solar Plexus Centering. Close your eyes and center your full attention on your central body region. Envision that inner region filled with light which radiates
throughout your body. Imagine the innermost part of your
body—deep within your chest and abdomen—bathed with
radiant light. Sense the release of tension as the light
expands to illuminate your total body—organs, systems,
joints, and muscles. Absorb the bright light deeper and
deeper into every cell of your body.

Step 2. Outer Illumination. Let the radiance permeating
your total body slowly expand, enveloping your full body
in an aura of bright energy. Envision the aura of energy
expanding and radiating outward.

Step 3. Cosmic Core Imagery. Envision the distant core
of the cosmos as a radiating dimension of light in its purest
form. Remind yourself that the cosmic energy core is the
cradle of all creation and the energizing source that sustains your existence.

Step 4. The Green Plane. Notice an expansive, iridescent
green plane reaching outward from the shining cosmic

core and radiating bright beams of energy in all directions throughout the universe.

Step 5. Energy Infusion. Turn the palms of your hands upward toward the green plane, and let its radiating beams of bright energy soak into your hands. Think of your hands as powerful receptors of cosmic energy. Sense the infusion of energy spreading from your hands to your solar plexus, and from there, throughout your body.

Step 6. Rejuvenation. Take a mental journey through your body by first scanning your body, beginning with your upper body region. As you progressively scan your body downward, bathe every cell and fiber with bright radiant energy. Target any problem area—a weak organ, dysfunctional system, or area of pain—and saturate it with bright, rejuvenating energy. Notice the warm, tingling, anti-aging energies flowing throughout your body.

Step 7. Balance. Upon completing the body scan, bring your hands together in a praying hands position to balance the infusion process and fully attune your mind, body, and spirit to the cosmic source of your existence. Affirm in your own words the rejuvenating results of the procedure.

Step 8. Reactivation. The rejuvenating effects of this procedure can be reactivated at any time through the following three-steps, which require only a few seconds (1) Turn your palms upward as you envision radiant green energy infusing your total body with rejuvenation; (2) use the praying-hands gesture to balance the new infusion of energy; and (3) affirm the powerful rejuvenating effects of the strategy.

Observations of the aura immediately following this procedure invariably reveal a brighter, more expansive aura along with the addition of shimmering, iridescent green. The addition can appear as a layer of color enveloping the full body, or it can appear as localized concentrations at particular body regions.

Summary

We now know that the higher cosmic dimension is not simply an impersonal reality, but rather a powerful aggregate of multiple planes and abundant growth resources. When we tap into those resources, the possibilities are simply unlimited. Each glimpse of the cosmic dimension expands our vision of ourselves and our place in the cosmos.

One of the great challenges we face in life is the discovery of new meaning to our existence. To overlook the cosmic dimension of our existence limits our search for meaning and severely constricts our growth. As a conscious life force, each of us is a work in progress—our evolution is clearly incomplete. Fortunately, all the resources we need to achieve our highest potentials are available to us now.

Chapter 6

Astral Projection and Rejuvenation

Astral projection, also known as out-of-body experience (OBE) and soul travel, is a state of awareness in which the locus of perception shifts to result in a conscious sense of being in a spatial location outside or away from the physical body.

The concept of astral projection is based on the *duality principle* of human nature, which holds that our basic makeup consists of both a biological body and a nonbiological counterpart. Although our biological and nonbiological parts are intimately linked, the nonbiological part, called the *astral body,* can temporarily separate from the physical body, and in that disengaged state, consciously experience other realities.

As a fully functional entity, the astral body, while in the projected state, remains connected to the physical body by a life-support system sometimes called the *silver cord.* The silver cord can span the far reaches of tangible as well as nontangible reality. It remains intact until our transition at death to the discarnate dimension. Once the silver cord is finally severed, the astral body is liberated to ascend to the discarnate realm of continued growth and fulfillment. According to many health care professionals, the astral body at the moment of death is often seen as a glowing mist gently rising above the physical body.

Except for physical baggage, nothing is lost at death. As we noted earlier, even that growth which was lost due to aging, disease, and injury is instantly regained at the moment of our transition to the other side. Incredibly, all the accumulated experiences of past lives are retained, conscious identity remains intact, and the liberated astral being instantly assumes the peak of all past development. From that peak, it is poised for even higher levels of enlightenment and astral actualization.

Out-of-body experiences are probably far more common than generally believed. They can range from simple awareness of being momentarily outside the body to extensive travel to distant places and other dimensions. During hypnosis, sensations of floating or drifting away from the physical body are common, particularly at deeper stages of the trance state. That spontaneous sense of being out of the body can include awareness of being suspended over the physical body as well as travel beyond immediate surroundings to experience spatially distant realities. Not infrequently, hypnotized subjects will describe traveling into outer space and viewing the earth from a distance.

Occasionally, surgical patients report having experienced OBEs during surgery. They describe rising above the body and viewing from overhead complex surgical procedures. In many instances, physicians have verified the accuracy of the patient's descriptions, which were often highly detailed and beyond the patient's expected knowledge of the procedures.

Analysis of dream journals suggests that OBEs are common during sleep. Examples are experiences of being borne aloft, viewing familiar terrain from above, and traveling to spatially distant locations. These experiences often include meaningful interactions with other people, some of whom were also in the out-of-body state. Interactions with departed loved ones, angels, and ministering guides are not unusual during the dream state.

OBEs often include remarkably detailed astral observations of higher cosmic planes. OBEs can break interdimensional barriers and facilitate direct interactions with other dimensions. They can access totally new sources of power and knowledge. They can probe the discarnate zone and provide us with a deeper understanding of life after death.

Fortunately, astral projection, while often spontaneous in nature, can be deliberately induced. Through mastery of appropriate procedures, we can generate the out-of-body state on command and focus the experience on certain desired outcomes. For instance, procedures are now available for using the out-of-body state to control pain, promote healing, facilitate learning, increase self-esteem, and overcome depression. (See my book *Astral Projection and Psychic Empowerment* for a detailed discussion of procedures related to these and other applications.)

Only recently have we developed procedures that use the out-of-body state to alter the aging process. But already, astral projection is considered a rejuvenation superstar. OBEs can tap dormant rejuvenation resources, including anti-aging energy, and directly generate a biological-astral balance, which is an essential element of rejuvenation.

Although the astral realm remains largely a mystery, astral projection gives us at the least a small glimpse of its wondrous possibilities. Analysis of OBEs of various age groups almost always reveals some reference to the rejuvenation effects of the experience. "Energized," "revitalized," "refreshed," "strengthened," "empowered," "restored," and "rejuvenated" are among the terms most frequently used. Also, descriptions of the accompanying presence of ministering guides throughout the experience are not unusual. Another common feature, particularly among reports that noted rejuvenation results, are impressions of literally traveling to a higher cosmic dimension of bright, rejuvenating energy.

There is considerable evidence to suggest that simply resting in the out-of-body state, independent of any effort to direct the experience, is healthful and rejuvenating. Our laboratory studies at Athens State University found that a period of only thirty minutes in the out-of-body state significantly increased strength of hand grip as measured by a hand dynamometer and dramatically expanded corona-discharge activity as recorded by electrophotography, both measures of which are associated with rejuvenation. With the introduction of structured out-of-body rejuvenation procedures, both strength of grip and corona-discharge activity increased even further. Our long-term studies of astral projection showed these indicators continued to increase until they eventually peaked where they then remained constant for the remainder of the studies.

Our research participants of all ages experienced during the out-of-body state a sense of command of the aging process, including a firm belief that they could slow aging and extend their life expectancies beyond the conventional limits. They began to see OBEs as powerful instruments of rejuvenation, which they could use to eliminate the effects of aging and improve the quality of their lives. Many of them began to perceive an unlimited life expectancy as not unrealistic. Upon the conclusion of our studies, our research participants were so convinced of the rejuvenation effects of astral projection that they continued to use the strategy regularly.

The ultimate astral rejuvenation plan establishes a powerful interaction between the biological body and its astral double. Once that interaction is established, awareness of higher astral dimensions through astral travel tends to strengthen the interaction and increase its rejuvenation effects. With the interaction firmly established and consciousness raised to a new level, the flow of anti-aging energy within the body tends to reach its peak. But like the physical body's nutritional needs, our rejuvenation needs are cyclic in nature. The powerful surge of rejuvenation resulting from astral projection is usually followed by a slow depletion of energy, thus requiring periodic repetition of the strategy. Although the rejuvenation effects of OBEs can be profound, the systematic integration of other rejuvenation options, including any of those we have already discussed, can help maintain a continuous flow of healthful, anti-aging energy.

In our laboratory, we researched numerous OBEs procedures in an effort to identify critical elements and principles related to successful induction and travel. Our studies revealed:

- A single "ideal" astral projection procedure is improbable due to the wide-ranging differences in abilities, attitudes, and expectations among individuals. Case studies of astral travelers revealed wide-ranging differences in procedures and techniques.

- Four critical elements characterize the most highly successful OBEs induction approaches. They are (1) motivation, (2) a success orientation, (3) appropriate imagery, and (4) positive affirmations. The four critical elements related to successful induction of the out-of-body state are likewise critical in achieving the goals of astral projection, including rejuvenation.

- The four critical elements characterizing successful OBEs do not constitute, in and of themselves, the out-of-body state. They are, however, essential means to an end. The first two elements—motivation and success orientation—are essential preliminary conditions. The second two elements—visualization and affirmation—are integrated into step-by-step procedures designed to generate the out-of-body state, promote astral travel, and facilitate achievement of important goals.

- As a general rule, the more flexible the induction procedure, the greater its effectiveness, not only in generating the out-of-body state, but in achieving the stated empowerment goals as well.

- The most effective affirmations are stated positively and informally, that is, in your own words, but within the framework of clearly formulated objectives.

In the following discussion, we will explore several out-of-body procedures specifically designed to promote rejuvenation. The step-by-step procedures are flexible, and can be easily modified to fit your personal needs, preferences, and comfort zone. The eyes are closed for each procedure, which requires approximately one hour. Each procedure should be conducted in a comfortable, quiet setting free of all distractions. Any interruption can abort the altered state and counteract its potential rejuvenation effects.

Each of the procedures presented here includes certain preliminaries. Among them are imagery of being enveloped in bright astral light along with invocations of astral guidance for the duration of the experience. You may also wish to invoke the presence of your personal ministering guide(s). Although some astral travels consider these invocations unnecessary, they are, nevertheless, relevant because they can facilitate productive travel and significantly enrich the astral experience.

Strategy 21

Astral Plane Procedure

The Astral Plane Procedure is based on the simple premise that, during the out-of-body state, we experience an elegant, intangible astral plane of incredible power. By lingering in that state, we can access pure astral energy which can, in turn, be deliberately transferred to the physical body at rest, using the silver cord as an energy transfer medium. Here is the procedure.

Step 1. Preliminaries. In a safe, comfortable, quiet place, settle back into a reclining position with your arms resting at your sides. In your own words, invoke astral guidance while envisioning yourself enveloped in bright astral light.

Step 2. Induction. To induce the out of body state, reach outward and hold the out-stretched position. As your arms become increasingly heavy, affirm in your own words that you are now prepared to slip out of your body. Now relax your arms and let them fall very slowly. Once your arms are finally at rest, sense yourself becoming so light that you begin to rise from your body. Let the process continue until you sense yourself fully suspended over your body. Take plenty of time for out-of-body awareness to emerge.

Step 3. Astral Awareness. Once securely out of your body, observe your physical body resting passively below, and the silver cord connecting you to it, typically at the abdominal or solar plexus region. Sense the bright, shimmering energy of astral space fully enveloping you and filling your astral body until you overflow with magnificent new power. Notice your complete sense of well-being and renewal. Take time to relish the splendor of this moment.

Step 4. Energy Transfer. Turn you attention again to your physical body at rest and the silver cord connecting you to it. Let the overflow of shining energy enveloping you surge forth into the silver cord and into your physical body. Let the profusion of pure astral energy saturate you physical body completely. Notice the bright glow of new, revitalizing energy enveloping your physical body. Allow plenty of time for the physical signs of aging to fade in the powerful glow of astral energy.

Step 5. Return. At this step, you can remain in the astral plane until you spontaneously return to your physical body, or you can deliberately initiate the return by centering your awareness on your physical body and giving yourself permission to return to it. Once reunited with your body, notice such physical sensations as warmth, tingling, and so forth, each of which signals an end to the out-of-body state.

Step 6. Conclusion. Before opening your eyes, take a few moments to review the out-of-body experience and its effects, both physical and mental. Notice especially the wondrous sense of physical and mental renewal. Conclude the procedure by affirming your power to access the astral realm and draw rejuvenating energy from it.

As with most rejuvenation strategies, the effectiveness of this procedure is increased through practice. Although many subjects find that they can induce a profound out-of-body state in a single trial using this procedure, others will require considerable practice to develop their skills, not only to enter the out-of-body state, but also to fully use its rejuvenation capacities.

Strategy 22

Astral Rejuvenation Through Hand Levitation

Another excellent OBEs induction and rejuvenation procedure is Astral Rejuvenation Through Hand Levitation. This procedure is an adaptation of hand levitation as used to induce self-hypnosis. Once the out-of-body state is achieved, step-by-step rejuvenation strategies are introduced. Here is the procedure.

Step 1. Preliminaries. Settle back into a relaxed, reclining position with your hands resting comfortably on your thighs. In your own words, invoke astral guidance while envisioning yourself enveloped in bright astral light.

Step 2. Relaxation. Take in a few deep breaths, exhaling slowly and pausing briefly between breaths. As you soak in the fresh air, notice the relaxation, first in your chest and then spreading slowly downward throughout your body. Let all tension leave your body as your breathing becomes slow, rhythmic, and effortless.

Step 3. Sensate Focusing. Focus your full attention on your hands at rest on your thighs. Notice each sensation—weight, warmth or coolness, pressure, moisture in your palms, texture of your clothing, and so forth. Next center your full attention on your right hand. Note the various sensations in that hand alone, paying particular attention to the weight of your hand and the pressure of your fingertips against your thigh.

Step 4. Hand Levitation. Continue to focus your full attention on your right hand, particularly the fingertips against your thigh. After a few moments, envision a glowing light form in the palm of your hand, gently pushing it upward. Notice the lightness, first spreading throughout your hand and then upward into your wrist and arm. Let your hand become increasingly light as you continue to sense the bright form in your palm, gently pushing your hand upward. Let your hand rise gently until it finally touches your forehead. Allow plenty of time for your hand to levitate. If at any point your hand resists or begins to fall, envision again the bright, luminous form in your palm gently pushing it upward.

Step 5. Out-of-Body State. Once your hand reaches your forehead, envision the light form in your palm spreading into your forehead and then enveloping your full body. Notice the sensation of lightness first felt in your hand now spreading throughout your body.

With your hand touching your forehead, give yourself permission to slide gently our of your body by simply relaxing your hand and letting it fall slowly downward. Once your hand comes to rest, sense yourself gently slipping out of your body. Your can facilitate that process by envisioning your astral body as a luminous form slowly rising above your physical body.

Step 6. Astral Rejuvenation. With your astral body now comfortably suspended over your physical body, sense the freedom and power of the moment. Think of your astral body as a spiritual copy of your physical body, and let yourself become totally infused with the rejuvenating light of the astral realm. Sense the renewal process as it permeates and revitalizes every fiber of your astral being.

Step 7. Physical Rejuvenation. As you remain suspended over your physical body, let the radiant glow of rejuvenation enveloping your astral body slowly expand until it fully envelops your physical body below. Take plenty of time for the astral-biological infusion of rejuvenating energy to reach its peak.

Step 8. The Return. Give yourself permission to return effortlessly to your physical body, taking with you the bright rejuvenating energies of the astral realm. As your are drawn gently into your physical body, let the accumulation of astral light permeate every biological organ and system, bathing them with bright astral energy. Now reunited with your physical body, note your sense of complete oneness with the cosmos.

Step 9. Cosmic Reflection. Review the out-of-body experience and reflect on its mental, physical, and spiritual effects. You may feel moved at this final step to express gratitude for the multiple benefits of the experience.

The energizing effects of this procedure are usually immediate and profound. The physical body takes on a youthful radiance that can linger for many hours, a phenomenon that can be objectively observed in the laboratory setting using electrophotographic procedures. Aside from its rejuvenating effects, this procedure is also relaxing and exhilarating. Many professionals, from politicians to performing artists, have used this procedure to energize them in preparation for an important presentation or performance. In the clinical setting, the procedure can be used in the treatment of depression and a variety of anxiety conditions.

Strategy 23

Destination Travel

Destination Travel is an out-of-body procedure designed to promote a state of general empowerment. When practiced regularly, the procedure generates a positive, optimistic state of mind, a condition that is critical to rejuvenation. It effectively takes the edge off of stress and induces a tranquil, relaxed state. It is especially recommended at times of crisis involving serious career demands, complicated personal relationships, unresolved conflicts, and perplexing spiritual issues. Here is the procedure.

Step 1. Preliminaries. Settle back, take in a few deep breaths, and develop a comfortable, effortless breathing pattern. In your own words, invoke astral guidance while envisioning yourself enveloped in bright astral light.

Step 2. Induction. Clear your mind of all active thought, and with your eyes closed, focus only on your breathing for a few moments. Shift your attention to the innermost part of yourself, and envision that part as a bright light form. Let that glowing form gently rise above your body, taking on in light-form the dimensions of your physical body, and transporting with it your conscious awareness. Take plenty of time for this process to unfold. Once the light-form embodying consciousness is suspended over your physical body, observe your body at rest below for a few moments. Stay with that external locus of awareness until you have firmly established a clear sense of being out of your physical body. Remind yourself that you are secure and protected by all the positive forces of the universe.

Step 3. Destination Control. As you remain out-of-body, select a favorite place—perhaps a safe retreat or a carefree setting from childhood with its rich memories—and give yourself permission to go there. Hold the clear image of your destination firmly in your mind until your experience the full reality of being there. (Note: This step is based on the concept that, in the out-of-body state, imagery combined with intent generates the essential vehicle for travel to selected destinations, whether on this earth plane or at some distant point in the cosmos.)

Step 4. Renewal. Having reached your destination, view your surroundings, and notice your sense of pleasure and personal fulfillment. Breathe in the wondrous energies enveloping you. Let the infusion of energy continue until you are totally energized and at your peak of full renewal.

Step 5. Goal Attainment. Envision your personal goals and affirm them in your own words as realities—either works in progress or already fulfilled. For rejuvenation, first envision yourself at your youthful prime, and then affirm your capacity to physically manifest that vision. For other goals, regardless of how varied they may be, envision them as realities—present or future—and affirm your power to experience them.

Step 6. The Return. To return to your physical body, turn your attention again to your body at rest, and give yourself permission to reunite with it. Upon re-entering your body, notice your physical sensations—breathing, heartbeat, body weight, and so forth—as signals of your return.

Step 7. Self-Empowerment Affirmations. With your astral and biological bodies now reunited, briefly review your out-of-body experience, and in your own words, affirm its empowering effects. Examples are: *Bright, rejuvenating energy is now flowing throughout my total being. I am infused with youthful vitality. I am at my peak—mentally, physically, and spiritually. I am fully empowered to achieve my personal goals of* (state goals).

Step 8. Postprocedure Cue. Conclude the procedure with the affirmation that simply envisioning the out-of-body destination selected for this procedure, and yourself interacting with it, is sufficient to instantly reactivate the procedure's empowerment effects.

For this procedure, the out-of-body travel destination can vary from session to session. As a general rule, the rejuvenation results seem to be greatest when the destination relates to youth. For self-improvement goals, out-of-body visits to settings of natural beauty, such as the seashore, a waterfall, or a mountain retreat, are excellent. For enlightenment goals, destinations involving higher cosmic dimensions, which can include interactions with ministering guides, often result in profound personal insight and spiritual enlightenment.

Strategy 24

Super Cosmic Highway

The Super Cosmic Highway is a procedure based on our case studies of astral travelers who reported a wide range of rejuvenation results. The procedure recognizes the importance of other dimensions beyond our known physical reality. Together, they offer a limitless array of invaluable benefits, including enlightenment, healing, and rejuvenation. Of equal or greater importance are the intelligent astral entities, particularly growth specialists and ministering guides, who are readily available to us.

Through our interactions with higher cosmic dimensions, we can reach beyond the constrictions of our present realities to enrich our lives with exciting new growth and understanding. Only then can we realize our highest potentials and achieve our loftiest goals. Although they beckon our awareness and interaction, we are, unfortunately, all too often alienated from them and their vast array growth resources.

The Super Cosmic Highway is designed to facilitate an empowering interaction with the cosmic realm as the highest source of rejuvenating energy. It recognizes the importance of astral projection as both an anti-aging strategy as well as an interactive vehicle for travel to the cosmic realm. The procedure includes the option (Step 5) of interacting with higher plane teachers and guides. Here is the full procedure.

Step 1. Preliminaries. Settle back into a comfortable, reclining or prone position, and with your eyes closed, give yourself permission to leave your body and travel to higher astral realms of energy. As you visualize yourself enveloped in bright astral light, affirm in your own words that cosmic escorts for the duration of the out-of-body experience will guide you.

Step 2. Induction. To induce the out-of-body state, first envision a higher cosmic dimension of pure light with a stream of bright energy forming a super highway that links you to the cosmic realm. As you continue to envision the super highway, sense the stream of pure cosmic energy entering your solar plexus and illuminating your total being. Let yourself become increasingly saturated with luminous energy. Once you are fully infused with cosmic energy, sense yourself gently rising from your body and entering upon the super highway of pure cosmic light.

Step 3. Cosmic Travel. With your astral being now safely situated on the cosmic highway, let yourself flow with the energy as you are drawn higher and higher toward its central light source. Continue to flow with the energy until your are finally enveloped in a higher cosmic dimension of bright light. Sense the wondrous infusion of unadulterated, rejuvenating energy. Enjoy the luxury of bathing in pure cosmic light.

Step 4. Energy Transfer. Turn your attention to the super cosmic highway connecting the cosmic dimension of energy to your physical body at rest in the distance. Let the highway become a functional conduit for the transfer of powerful rejuvenating energy. From your position in the cosmic realm, let the transfer of energy continue until an expansive aura of bright cosmic energy fully envelops your body resting comfortably at a distance.

Step 5 (Optional). As you linger in the cosmic realm, you can increase its rejuvenating and enlightening effects by interacting with the dimension's ministering specialists. These are advanced cosmic teachers and guides who are always available to share their resources and guide our growth. Through them, you can discover the personal side of cosmic planes. At this stage, astral travelers often discover an astral entity that becomes a long-term personal guide.

Step 6. The Return. To reunite with your physical body, give yourself permission to return by simply flowing with the energy being transferred on the super cosmic highway to your physical body. Once reunited with your body, typically within a few seconds, notice various physical sensations, such as tingling, breathing, and heartbeat, all of which signal your safe return to your body.

Step 7. Rejuvenation Augmentation. Now reunited with your physical body, notice the rejuvenating cosmic energy flowing throughout your being. You can augment the rejuvenating effects of the experience by focusing on various body regions, organs, and systems, and mentally saturating them with bright energy. Pay particular attention to restoring damaged tissue, opening blocked systems, and bathing malfunctioning organs. Turn your attention to the outward signs of aging and mentally disperse bright cosmic energy over your outer body. Again, use imagery and positive affirmations to smooth away wrinkles, lift and revitalize sagging muscles, and impart a youthful glow over your full body.

Step 8. Conclusion and Postprocedure Cue. Briefly review and reaffirm in your own words the empowering effects of the experience. End the experience with the following postprocedure cue: *By simply envisioning the beam of light connecting me to the cosmic source of power, I can activate personal empowerment and rejuvenation— mental, physical, and spiritual—at any moment.*

Aside from rejuvenation, the Super Cosmic Highway has many other important empowerment applications. An increased sense of well-being and personal control over one's life almost always accompanies the procedure, especially when it includes the optional Step 5.

In the clinical setting, the procedure has shown great promise in the treatment of various disorders, including obsessive-compulsive conditions and phobias. It has also been highly effective in the treatment for chronic pain. With repeated use of the procedure as a pain management strategy, many patients experienced complete recovery from chronic pain along with marked improvements in their general health status.

In the academic setting, students who had practice the procedure and then used the postprocedure cue immediately prior to important examinations or classroom presentations reported significant improvement in their performance. They reported greater self-confidence, less anxiety, and a marked improvement in memory.

Strategy 25

Emerald Cord Procedure

As discussed in a previous chapter, cosmic planes exist in an array of colors, with each color signifying the plane's empowerment specialty. The white plane is an all-purpose plane—interacting with it, as expected, can have multiple benefits. Planes of color, on the other hand, are highly concentrated planes of specialized energy. As a general rule, the brighter the plane, the higher the concentration of energy. The blue plane is associated with balance and cosmic attunement; the yellow plane is associated with learning and intellectual growth; and the violet plane is associated with spiritual enlightenment and self-actualization. The iridescent emerald plane is known for its high concentration of rejuvenating and healing energy. Many other planes of different colors and related specialties exist throughout the cosmos. Planes of several mixed colors, sometimes called rainbow planes, possess the combined empowerment attributes of each color. (For a further discussion of multiple cosmic planes and their empowerment specialties, see *Astral Projection and Psychic Empowerment.*)

The bright emerald plane is one of the most readily accessible planes in the cosmos, and its valuable properties are highly responsive to human interaction. Its healing and rejuvenating resources can be readily transferred to this reality dimension, often in a visible form that can be seen entering the physical body's surrounding energy fields during the astral state. Out-of-body travelers to the emerald plane often compare its iridescent coloration to the emerald gem, which is also valued by many for its rejuvenation properties. Tending to confirm the anti-aging effects of this gem is its popularity among centenarians as discussed later in this book.

The Emerald Cord Procedure is structured to access the emerald plane and actually transport its healthful, rejuvenating energy to the physical body during the out-of-body state. The procedure, while focusing on rejuvenation of the physical body, is also designed to rejuvenate the astral body as the energizing medium.

The Emerald Cord Procedure recognizes the "silver cord" as a functional, pliant link connecting the projected astral body to its physical body counterpart. In the projected astral state, the "silver cord" serves not only a critical support function—it also becomes a functional channel for the transfer of powerful cosmic energy.

This procedure recognizes the capacity of the astral body to ascend as a transient traveler to the highest realms in the cosmos. Through astral travel, we can access the same cosmic energies that will be available to us after our final transition to the other side. Here is the procedure.

Step 1. Induction. Induce the out-of-body state by following Steps 1 and 2 of Destination Travel as previously presented.

Step 2. Cosmic Scan. Take a few moments to scan the vast cosmos from your projected position. With limitless astral vision, notice the cosmic core of pure light along with distant planes, forms, and dimensions. Remind yourself that, in the astral state, you are protected and secure. All the higher energies of the cosmos are now available to you. You can be wherever you decide to be.

Step 3. Cosmic Travel to the Emerald Plane. Locate the luminous emerald plane in the distance and focus your full attention upon it. Give yourself permission to travel to it, letting yourself be drawn gently into its energy field. Allow plenty of time for your astral body to merge with the luminous, rich green plane. Bathed in the bright plane's powerful energy, let your astral body become fully infused until it overflows with rejuvenation. With your mental and spiritual functions at their peaks, linger for a few moments in the powerful glow of this plane, and let new insights and creative solutions emerge spontaneously.

Step 4. Rejuvenation Transfer. As the emerald plane's energy continues to fully infuse your astral body, shift your attention to the silver cord connecting you to your physical body at rest in the distance. Let the emerald plane's bright energy pour into the cord, transforming its silvery energy to shining green. Allow the iridescent green energy flowing through the silver cord to finally reach your physical body, bathing and saturating it with verdant rejuvenation. Let the energy transfer process continue until you are totally infused with rejuvenation—mentally, physically, and spiritually. You will sense when the infusion process is complete.

Step 5. The Return. Give yourself permission to return to your physical body resting in the distance. You will sense yourself being drawn to your body and gently being reunited with it. Once the re-engagement is complete, focus your attention on your breathing and various other physical sensations.

Step 6. Conclusion. Review the experience, and reflect on its rejuvenating effects. Sense the youthful energy flowing throughout your physical body.

Our laboratory studies designed to identify the physiological effects of this procedure indicated lower blood pressure and slower pulse rate immediately following the procedure. Electrophotographic measures, sometimes called aura photography, indicated brighter and significantly expanded corona discharge activity, along with regions of luminous green coloration, patterns that tended to persist for several days following application of this procedure.

Aside from its primary usefulness as a rejuvenation strategy, the Emerald Cord Procedure has been remarkably effective in stimulating creativity. College students whose majors included art, music, and journalism report having discovered totally new concepts and motifs through out-of-body travel to the emerald plane. Of particular note was a psychology graduate student who used the procedure to generate a highly innovative dissertation proposal, which met the solid approval of her doctoral committee.

Strategy 26

Cosmic Fountain of Youth

Many astral travelers report spontaneous visitations to a distant cosmic fountain of rejuvenating energy. From their descriptions, we devised the Cosmic Fountain of Youth, a procedure based on the premise that there exists not one but two fountains of youth—the one within yourself and the other in the outer cosmos. The procedure guides astral travel to the fountain where the astral body is bathed in a sparkling spray of rejuvenating energy. The procedure energizes and balances the inner fountain of youth with the outer cosmic fountain of unlimited rejuvenation. Here is the procedure.

Step 1. Induction. Induce the out-of-body state by following Steps 1 and 2 of Destination Travel as previously presented.

Step 2. Cosmic Travel. As you remain out of body, view the cosmos with its many planes, pathways, and other forms. Search the cosmos until you discover a brilliant bluish-green energy plane. Give yourself permission to engage the plane, and upon entering it, let yourself be drawn to its innermost region where you will discover a sparkling fountain with its arching spray of bright energy. Allow plenty of time for you to engage the plane and its innermost region. Once comfortably in the presence of the plane's fountain, enter the fountain's spray and let its streams of invigorating energy bathe your astral body. Sense rejuvenating energy rising from your inner fountain of youth, then merging with the outer fountain's spray of rejuvenating energy. Let the inner and outer merging of energy continue until your inner fountain becomes totally energized, balanced, and attuned to the outer cosmic fountain of abundant energy.

Step 3. The Return. With your inner fountain now fully functional and completely energized, step from the fountain and turn your attention to your physical body at rest. Give yourself permission to return to your physical body and reunite with it. Upon merging with your physical body, sense the powerful infusion of cosmic energy rejuvenating every fiber, muscle, joint, and tendon of your body. Sense the wear and tear effects of stress and aging gently dissolving away. Your total body is revitalized and fortified with powerful, rejuvenating energy. As the dynamic energy drawn from your inner fountain and the outer cosmic fountain blend and surge throughout your physical body, you can sense the warm restoration of youth and vigor.

Step 4. Conclusion. End the procedure by envisioning both your inner fountain of youth and the outer sparkling cosmic fountain. Bring your hands together as a gesture of your oneness with the two fountains and the powerful merging within yourself of inner and outer rejuvenating energy.

This procedure is one of the most effective strategies known for inducing a state of inner balance and attunement with the universe, conditions that alone are rejuvenating. Add to these a direct access to the highest source of rejuvenating energy and the possibilities are simply unlimited. Arresting aging and reversing its effects, revitalizing physical organs and systems, and totally renewing the mind and body are all within your reach when your tap into the inner and outer fountains of youth.

Summary

Astral projection is one of the most important human growth channels known. In that state, all the faculties of human consciousness remain intact, and in some instances, they are actually liberated to a higher level of efficiency. Out-of-body perceptions are often clearer, cognitive functions more complex, and creative processes more advanced. Liberated from the constrictions of biological experience, conscious awareness is unleashed to experience new realities and interact with other dimensions. By mastering this important phenomenon, we can dramatically accelerate our growth, rejuvenate the mind and body, and achieve a higher level of personal growth and self-realization. Possibly more than any other human experience, OBEs manifest the continuity and permanence of our existence as a conscious life force.

Also see my book *Astral Projection and Psychic Empowerment* for a further discussion of the empowerment possibilities of astral projection.

Chapter 7

Rejuvenation and the Human Aura

The human aura is an integral component of the self's larger energy system. As a colorful energy field enveloping the physical body, the aura is an external energy phenomenon emanating from an inner energy core which is, in turn, our link to the higher cosmic source of our existence. The external aura along with its inner core, which is believed to be situated in the body's solar plexus region, constitutes a unique energy system that is intrinsically cosmic and indestructible in nature. It is our connection to the infinite power of the universe. When attuned to the higher dimensions of energy, the aura and its energizing core are a source of unlimited insight, power, and knowledge.

The aura system is the essential energy force without which we would not exist. As a manifestation of the cosmic source of life, the aura system energies every fiber of our being, both in this life and life on the other side. All our past lifetimes, as well as our existence in the discarnate intervals between them, were energized by it.

The external aura provides a visible index to our past and present growth. Each individual aura is typically characterized by a dominant color and unique structural features that constitute the individual's so-called *aura signature*. All our past development along with our current mental, physical, emotional, social, and spiritual characteristics are registered in the aura. Fortunately, we can acquire effective strategies for viewing the aura and intervening directly into the aura system.

The aura system is relevant to rejuvenation in a variety of ways. The constricted aura, which is often associated with stress and blocked growth, depletes our energy resources, and thereby contributes to aging. The unbalanced aura, which is often associated with conflict and frustration, impairs the functioning of critical biological organs, and thereby contributes to aging. The discolored aura, which is often associated with depression and chronic fatigue, exhausts the aura system, and thereby contributes to aging. Finding ways of enriching the aura and using its growth potentials is therefore critical to our personal development, and more specifically, to rejuvenation.

A healthy, functional aura system is essential to our mental, physical, and spiritual well-being. By intervening into the dysfunctional aura system, we can introduce changes that strengthen the aura and accelerate our growth. Advanced strategies that access the aura's central core can balance the aura and attune it to our cosmic origins while enabling us to maximize our potentials and achieve our highest goals.

Highly advanced rejuvenation approaches almost always recognizes the indispensable role of the aura. Fortunately, the aura system can be readily incorporated into structured procedures, which either use its rejuvenation potentials or enhance its various functions. A bright, balanced, attuned aura is an essential component of any comprehensive rejuvenation plan. To overlook the anti-aging potentials of the aura would seriously limit our rejuvenation efforts. In the following discussion, we will explore several strategies designed specifically to activate the aura's anti-aging capacities.

Strategy 27

Aura Hand-Viewing Strategy

Although aura rejuvenation strategies do not always require actually viewing the aura, an effective self-viewing strategy can be useful in determining the aura's characteristics and needs, as well as the effects of our rejuvenation efforts. But aside from the assessment side of aura viewing, simply viewing the aura, whether one's own aura or that of another person, is almost always relaxing, energizing, and rejuvenating.

Among the most effective self-viewing techniques is the Aura Hand-viewing Strategy, a procedure that requires only seconds to implement. As with most viewing techniques, natural or indirect lighting and a neutral or off-white background are recommended for this strategy. The procedure first generates an optical illusion called the "white-out effect" which is then replaced by the visible aura. It is important to note that the glowing white-out effect is not the aura but rather an illusion that precedes the emergence of the visible aura. Here is the Aura Hand-viewing Strategy.

Step 1. Hand Gaze. Hold your hand at arm's length, and gaze for a few moments at your hand with fingers slightly spread.

Step 2. Peripheral Vision. While gazing at your hand, slowly expand your peripheral vision to take in your total visual field.

Step 3. White-Out Effect. Once your peripheral vision reaches its limits, let your eyes fall slightly out-of-focus. You will immediately notice a milky white glow called the "white-out effect" enveloping your hand.

Step 4. Aura View. Gaze at the glow around your hand until the aura with its colors and patterns comes into view, typically within a few seconds. Notice the relaxing and energizing effects that accompany the viewing experience.

Because the aura surrounding the hand is similar in many ways to the aura enveloping the total body, the Aura Hand-viewing Strategy is highly useful as a pre- and posttest procedure in determining the effects of rejuvenation strategies designed to influence the aura. Furthermore, viewing the aura at the beginning of a procedure prepares us mentally to engage the aura and intervene into its functions. Also, viewing the aura at the end of a procedure increases the rejuvenation effectiveness of the procedure. Fortunately, the aura, while relatively stable, is highly receptive to even mild empowerment efforts. The most highly effective rejuvenation strategy will include aura viewing at the beginning and end of the procedure, along with in-between steps designed to promote a rejuvenated aura, which is typically expansive, bright, and balanced.

As a footnote, the Aura Hand-viewing Strategy, while designed to view one's own aura, can be easily revised for viewing the full aura of another person. For that application, gaze at the subject's forehead from a comfortable distance and gradually expand your peripheral vision. Upon reaching your peripheral limits, let your eyes fall slightly out of focus to induce the white-out effect. Gaze at the white glow surrounding your subject until the full aura with its colors and other features becomes visible, typically within a few seconds.

Strategy 28

Aura Conditioning Strategy

Just as physical exercise is critical to a healthy body, aura exercise is critical to a healthy aura. The Aura Conditioning Strategy is based on the premise that deliberately exercising the aura strengthens its health and rejuvenation properties. This high impact strategy introduces a sleek combination of controlled breathing and colorful imagery to generate a rhythmic pattern of aura expansion and contraction. The procedure is based on the following observations:

- Typically, deeply inhaling expands the aura whereas slowly exhaling contracts it.

- When appropriate imagery is introduced, the expansion-contraction process is intensified.

- Exercising the aura's expansion-contraction functions through appropriately controlled breathing fortifies the aura with bright new energy.

- The energized aura unleashes its rejuvenating properties to suppress the aging process and infuse the physical body with rejuvenation.

- Increased mental alertness and a heightened sense of well-being invariably accompany the aura energizing process.

- Regularly exercising the aura builds a strong aura system while cultivating its rejuvenation potentials.

Here is the procedure.

Step 1. Controlled Breathing. Settle back and center your full attention on your breathing. Take in a few deep breaths and exhale slowly as relaxation gently spreads throughout your body.

Step 2. Mental Imagery. Envision your aura rhythmically expanding as you inhale and contracting as you exhale. With each breath you take, sense the infusions of bright, new energy throughout your aura system—from its inner-most core to its outermost regions. (Note: You can observe the bright expansion-contraction process as it occurs in your aura by using the Aura Hand-viewing Strategy as previously discussed.)

Step 3. Deep Rejuvenation. With your aura now glowing with luminous rejuvenating energy, focus your attention on your aura's innermost core as it pulsates with new power. Intensify the rejuvenation process by deeply inhaling the bright energies of youth and slowly exhaling the dull residue of aging. Allow the brightness of your aura system to fully infuse your physical body, totally renewing it from the inside out. Envision specific body regions, organs, and systems, and mentally bathe them with bright, anti-aging energy. Take plenty of time for rejuvenating energy to saturate your total being—mentally, physically, and spiritually.

Step 5. Affirmation of Power. With rejuvenating energy now flowing deep within, conclude the procedure by affirming: *I am at my peak of rejuvenation and personal power.*

Strategy 29

Aura Rejuvenation Strategy

This strategy is specifically designed to activate on command the aura's rejuvenation functions. Designed primarily to infuse the aura with bright, rejuvenating energy, it typically expands the aura and increases the brilliance of aura colors. It effectively balances the aura and generates a highly attuned mental and physical state.

Step 1. Aura Viewing. View your aura using the Aura Hand-viewing Strategy as previously presented. Note particularly any dullness or constriction in the distribution of energy around your hand.

Step 2. Materialization of Light. Briskly rub your hands together to generate an accumulation of energy between then. Then, with your hands held at arm's length, palm against palm, slowly separate your hands by a few inches.

Cup your hands slightly and allow a bright, glowing sphere of concentrated energy to form between your palms, a phenomenon known as the "materialization of light."

Step 3. Cosmic Connection. Turn your hands upward with the sphere of energy in your palms. Envision bright energy from the distant core of the cosmos joining the sphere of energy in your palms. Sense the powerful accumulation of energy within your palms.

Step 4. Aura Self-Massage. Gently place the sphere of bright energy over your solar plexus region, and gently massage your aura at that region with circular hand motions while carefully avoiding any physical contact with the body.

Step 5. Energy Infusion. Let bright new energy spread deeply into your central energy region and then throughout your total aura system. Sense the powerful energy infusing your aura's inner core and then spreading outward to envelop your total body, literally dissolving away the external signs of aging. Let the infusion of new energy saturate your physical body as organs and systems are energized and renewed.

Step 6. Conclusion. Again, view your aura using the Aura Hand-viewing Strategy. Note the changes in your aura, particularly the increase in brightness and expansiveness. Affirm in your own words the rejuvenating results of the procedure.

Strategy 30

Aura Attunement Strategy

Like the bright, expansive aura, the attuned aura signifies rejuvenation and defies aging. Although the Aura Rejuvenation Strategy as discussed above tends to balance the aura's energy functions, a full attunement of the aura often requires a more focused effort that brings the aura's multiple functions into a state of total oneness. The Aura Attunement Strategy is designed to achieve that goal.

The procedure introduces the Aura Caress (Step 2), a technique that identifies disruptions in the aura's frequency patterns, and classifies the aura's current level of attunement within a range of one to seven. A level of one signals a weak, underdeveloped, or inefficient aura system; whereas a level of seven represents the ultimate aura system. Many aura specialists view the ultimate level of seven as reserved either for the discarnate realm, or else only temporarily reached during such phenomena as the peak experience. Although the Aura Caress was originally designed to measure the aura attunement levels of other persons, it is adapted here for self-use. While impressionistic in nature, it can provide an important diagnostic picture of the aura's current functions.

The Aura Attunement Strategy also introduces the Inner Aura Massage (Step 3). The typical aura has numerous spherical rims of energy, the outer of which conceivably extends to infinity. By massaging the innermost spherical rim, which is within a few inches of the physical body, we can generate a balanced, attuned state throughout the total aura. The result is symmetry among the auras various spheres within spheres, and a powerful release of the aura's rejuvenating resources.

Here is the full Aura Attunement Strategy, including the Aura Caress and Inner Aura Massage.

Step 1. Preliminaries. Find a quiet, comfortable place and set aside approximately thirty minutes for the procedure.

Step 2. Aura Caress. The Aura Caress is designed to measure the aura's current level of attunement, which ranges from a low of one to a high of seven. Prepare yourself for the procedure by settling back and clearing your mind of active thought. Focus your attention on your aura's energizing core situated in your solar plexus region. You can sense the core's powerful energies radiating outward by placing your hands, palm sides down, over your solar plexus at a few inches from your body. By moving your hands slowly away from your body, you will sense the intensity of the energy diminishing. To determine the nature of your aura's frequencies, lightly rest your left wrist, palm side down, in the palm of your right hand. Feel the weight and warmth of your wrist as it rests in your palm. Sense the interacting energies between your palm and wrist. Note any disturbance in the interaction, a phenomenon known as *auric static*. Notice the strength of the energy vibrations, and any unusual fluctuations in energy levels. To determine your current level of aura attunement, envision a small probe situated between your palm and wrist, and leading to an instrument device with a pointer and dial consisting of numbers one through seven. Allow the pointer to move across the dial and eventually stabilize at a number that represents your present level of attunement. Allow plenty of time for the pointer to stabilize.

Step 3. Inner Aura Massage. To begin the massage, envision your personal aura as a series of energy spheres within spheres enveloping your physical body. Next, rest your hands over your solar plexus region with palm sides down, while avoiding physical touch.

Slowly lift your hands until you sense warm, tingling sensations in your palms, a signal that you have reached the boundary of your aura's innermost sphere. With your palms remaining turned toward your body, gently stroke the outside boundary of the sphere, first horizontally and then vertically. Continue to stroke the frontal boundary of the sphere to evenly disperse its energy. Although the sphere encases your total body, by stroking only the sphere's frontal space, you can create a dynamic pattern of balanced energy that flows throughout the inner sphere and into the aura's outer regions.

Step 4. Cosmic Attunement. Turn your palms upward as you envision your total aura interacting with bright energy of cosmic origin. Sense the harmonious frequencies of pure cosmic energy interacting with your personal aura, further balancing and attuning it.

Allow the interaction to continue until you are fully attuned and energized with bright cosmic energy.

Step 5. Aura Caress. Repeat the Aura Caress as described in Step 2 above. Note the changes in your aura's frequency patterns and attunement level.

Strategy 31

Rejuvenation Replacement Therapy

Rejuvenation Replacement Therapy is a self-intervention strategy designed to replenish our inner reservoir of rejuvenation resources. Although any strategy that exercises our rejuvenation potentials tends to generates new anti-aging resources, a direct infusion of new energy is at times required.

A variety of life situations can deplete our rejuvenation resources. Common examples are excessive stress, physical illness, chronic pain, depression, conflict, personal loss, and insecurity. Rejuvenation Replacement Therapy, while not designed to directly resolve these issues, empowers us to cope more effectively with them. When we are infused with positive energy, we experience a new sense of personal power over conditions that could otherwise overwhelm us.

Aura Replacement Therapy focuses on the total aura system, including its powerful energizing core and its external components consisting of enveloping spheres within spheres of energy. Depletion of aura energy is seen as a malfunction of the inner core. The primary goal of the procedure is to jump-start the total aura system and fortify it with a powerful increase of new energy. Here is the procedure.

Step 1. Inner Aura Core. Settle back into a comfortable position, and with your eyes closed, envision your inner aura core as a glowing, pulsating orb with power to distribute energy throughout the aura enveloping your physical body.

Step 2. External Aura. Envision your external aura as a series of spheres within spheres of energy enveloping the physical body.

Step 3. Cosmic Energy System. Envision a cosmic core of limitless energy situated at the center of the universe, radiating energy in all directions to sustain and energize the total universe. Think of your own energy system with its core and surrounding energy as a replica of the cosmic energy system.

Step 4. Cosmic Congruency. Envision the outermost region of your aura system interfacing infinite energy of cosmic origin. Embrace the energy emanating from the center of the cosmos, and allow it to meld with your own energy system. Sense the integration of personal and cosmic energy, first in the external regions of your aura, and then throughout your total aura system.

Step 5. Energy Amplification. As your energy system interacts with the ultimate source of cosmic energy, sense the tremendous burst of rejuvenating cosmic energy in your aura's inner core, and then spreading progressively outward until your total aura is fully infused with new energy.

Strategy 32

Concentration and Transfer of Cosmic Energy

Once your aura system is adequately energized, you can generate a visible concentration of pure cosmic energy and transfer it to a specific body area that may need to be energized or renewed. This procedure is especially useful in fortifying weak or damaged physical organs and dysfunctional biological systems. Here is the procedure.

Step 1. Goal Formulation. Formulate your goals, to include identifying the specific biological region, function, or system to be energized.

Step 2. Energy Concentration. Bring your palms together and rub them briskly against each other. Upon sensing the buildup of energy between your palms, slowly separate them, and with your hands cupped, notice the ball of pure white energy suspended between your palms.

Step 3. Energy Transfer. Place the ball of cosmic energy at any designated body location, and gently massage it into the aura by using circular motions while carefully avoiding direct contact with the physical body, which can negate the transfer effort by scattering the energy. To energize a particular physical organ or body region, gently massage the ball of energy into the aura at that location. To rejuvenate a biological system, such as the cardiovascular, or to stimulate the rejuvenation process, place the ball of energy at your solar plexus region and gently massage it into the aura. To erase the external signs of aging, place the ball of energy at the area to be rejuvenated and gently massage it into the aura, again using circular motions and carefully avoiding physical touch. You can even energize the brain with this procedure by placing the ball of energy anywhere around the head region and gently massaging it into the aura.

Step 4. Aura Balancing and Attunement. Balance your aura system by again rubbing your hands together briskly and then touching your temples with your fingertips as you affirm: *I am fully balanced and attuned, both inwardly and outwardly.*

Step 5. Rejuvenation Cue: Hand Rub and Temple Touch. Tell yourself in your own words that by simply rubbing your hands together and touching your temples, you can reactivate rejuvenation of both mind and body.

This procedure has been used effectively by a wide range of age groups. In our studies, marked improvements in cognitive functions were noted when cosmic energy was massaged into the aura at the head region in Step 3. Memory improved rapidly for residents in a retirement facility following only limited practice of the procedure. College students who practiced the procedure likewise showed a significant increase in memory. The memory task for both groups required them to recall a series of digits as well as the contents of a paragraph that had been presented verbally to them. Intellectual functions, which included tasks requiring abstract thinking, also improved for both groups. During the evaluation sessions, it was noted that both groups frequently used the Hand Rub and Temple Touch technique as a rejuvenation cue (Step 5).

Social Interaction and Psychic Vampirism

Critical to the aura energy system and its functions are our interactions with others. Positive social interactions tend to energize and rejuvenate all that participate in the interaction. Interactions between two or more people who value and trust each other are particularly energizing. Because of the synergy effect, the energizing results for both participants are greater than anything that would have been possible for them individually. The synergistic effect of teamwork in often evident in competitive sports. A recent example is the 1999 U.S. Women's World Cup soccer team. Their interconnected teamwork clearly gave them the winning edge.

Romantic interactions between partners can be particularly rejuvenating. Observations of the aura during such interactions show a bright expansion of each aura and in some instances, a literal union of the two auras. Among the essential conditions that promote positive partner relationships and, in turn, contribute to a healthy, rejuvenated energy system, are (1) A genuine exchange of affection, understanding, and respect; (2) trust and security in the relationship; and (3) freedom to be oneself.

Unfortunately, personal interactions are not always positive and rejuvenating. Examples are interactions involving persons who do not value and trust each other. The result, over time, can be a serious depletion of the aura's reservoir of critical energy. Betrayal, deception, and disingenuous interactions are particularly detrimental—they negate the synergistic potential of any relationship.

Of even more serious consequence to the human energy system is the direct loss of energy associated with a phenomenon known as *psychic vampirism*. Because the consequences of psychic vampirism are so serious, along with the fact that psychic vampirism appears to be on the increase in our culture, we will explore in considerable depth the nature of this phenomenon and ways of counteracting it.

Psychic vampirism is a complex, interrelated phenomenon in which one's energies are transferred, usually involuntarily, to the psychic vampire whose strategies are mental instead of physical. Rather than grotesque villains who pounce on their prey and gorge on blood under cover of darkness, the psychic vampire is the unfortunate victim of a flawed energy system that is sustained only by the habitual consumption of energy from another human energy system. They invade the aura system of their host victim to meet their own energy deficiencies or to satisfy their aberrant drives, including their exaggerated needs to dominate, control, and in some instances, even destroy their host victims.

By feeding on the energies of others, the psychic vampire is temporarily rejuvenated and energized while the unsuspecting victim is left energy deficient, fatigued, and vulnerable. Not surprisingly then, observations of the victim's aura immediately following a vampire interaction consistently reveal a dull, constricted aura; whereas, the psychic vampire's aura assumes a temporarily bright expansiveness. In long-term vampire inter-actions, the victim becomes increasing deficient in critical health and rejuvenation resources while the vampire becomes increasingly dependent on the temporary "high" of instant energy infusions.

In contrast to the legendary vampire, psychic vampires possess no extraordinary powers. They are neither supernatural nor bizarre. They cannot materialize, vanish, or change into other creatures, and they do not defy gravity. They do not feed on their victims' blood, and they are not repelled by garlic or religious symbols. They are not adverse to sunlight, and their images are clearly visible in a mirror. They are found in a wide range of occupational settings—factories, retail stores, classrooms, government, churches and synagogues, and even hospitals. From the assembly line to the executive board room to the highest seats of government, psychic vampires are there, poised to exercise their vampire drives and prey on their unsuspecting victims. They can appear outwardly "normal" and even benevolent, but underneath they are typically agitated, insecure, and unstable. Deep down, they feel vulnerable and underappreciated. Inept and insecure, they often try to drag others down to their level. Case histories of psychic vampires revealed they were often cruel, barbaric, savage leaders in a past life who were responsible for great loss of lives. They were often oppressors of the weak, and many of them had achieved fame for their military feats. They were occasionally women rulers in a past life, seen as strong and powerful leaders.

Psychic vampirism, like its legendary counterpart, has a long and interesting history. Even the scriptural account of Adam and Eve suggests a unique vampire theme, with the taking of Adam's rib to create woman suggesting a transfer of not only biological tissue, but also life-sustaining energy. In another instance, Christ reported feeling the energy leave his body when a woman touched the hem of his garment.

The antithesis of psychic vampirism involving the positive transfer of energy is also suggested in the Bible. A case in point is the account of Christ restoring sight to a blind man through physical touch alone. Certain healing practices, such as the "laying-on-of-hands" as seen among certain contemporary religions, suggest a voluntary transfer of positive energy, either from the healer or a higher source. Psychic healing is sometimes explained as the transfer of healing energy from the psychic to the recipient. These examples reveal the empowering possibilities of the positive transfer of energy. The negative transfer of energy as seen in psychic vampirism, on the other hand, has no redeeming qualities—the results are detrimental to vampire and victim alike.

Often unevolved in their personal development, psychic vampires are driven by their need to survive, but having failed to develop their inner survival resources, they turn outward, and in desperation, take life-sustaining energy from others. But because the rewards of their compulsion are fleeting, psychic vampires often seek fulfillment through other channels in which their vampire traits are subtly disguised. In *sublimation,* for instance, the unacceptable vampire impulse is buried in the subconscious and then redirected through socially acceptable channels, such as fundraising (taking money rather than energy from others). In another disguise called *reaction formation,* the vampire impulse is subconsciously expressed through opposite and often extreme behaviors, such as large charitable gestures (giving rather than taking) or excessive-helping behaviors. Along another line, our studies of drug abuse often revealed underlying psychic vampire tendencies among abusers. Drugs, however, did not satisfy their energy needs—they continued to practice psychic vampirism.

In addition to these tactics, the vampire impulse can be expressed through exploitation, manipulation, and greed as well as an overwhelming drive for wealth, status, and recognition. But despite their efforts, personal fulfillment and empowerment elude the psychic vampire. Eventually, many of them end up loathing themselves and the victims of their vampire tactics. Unfortunately, they are often deficient in personal insight; and they seldom seek help in overcoming their self-defeating behaviors.

The underlying dynamic of psychic vampirism is, in some ways, analogous to certain other psychic phenomena. In *psychokinesis* (Pk), for instance, sheer mind power is focused on either internal or external targets in an effort to induce desired change, usually by bombarding them with positive energy. Given the power of the mind to target and send energy, it would follow that the mind's focusing efforts could be reversed to draw energy from external targets, including other people.

Telepathy, or mind to mind communication, further illustrates some of the dynamics associated with psychic vampirism. Telepathy reflects the capacity of the mind to mentally send and receive thought messages. A variation of telepathy is the capacity of the psychic mind to deliberately tap into the thought processes of others. Since thought itself is a type of energy, certain inappropriate forms of telepathy could border on psychic vampirism. Examples are telepathic processes that invade and feed on the thought functions of others.

It is important to emphasize here that, while psychic vampirism can draw energy directly from the host victims, telepathic efforts to adversely influence others by sending negative messages or energies are detrimental to the sender alone. Negative energies, once generated in the mind, are self-adhesive—they resist all efforts to send or transfer to others. They are, consequently, disempowering only to the person who generates and harbors them. Although psychic faculties, along with any other cognitive faculty, can be misused, psychic vampirism is one of the very few instances of psychic phenomena that is consistently detrimental to all involved. By invading another person's energy space, it disregards the rights of others and violates all normal expectations of human interaction.

The energy transaction between psychic vampire and victim is often spontaneous, and may in fact occur subconsciously for both participants. Even when the vampire transaction is complete, the victim, unaware that an energy transfer has occurred, may attribute the loss of energy and ensuing fatigue to other factors. From the psychic vampire's perspective, the energy infusion process may be perceived simply as a rewarding or enriching social interaction.

Although psychic vampirism can be spontaneous and subconscious, it is often intentionally initiated by the vampire who stealthily taps into the energy system of selected victims. The unsuspecting victims of such interactions are all too often vulnerable and defenseless. When the interaction is frequent and long-term, the consequences can be devastating. Chronic fatigue, increased risk of serious illness, accelerated aging, and depression are among the results. While the exact incidence of such interactions is unknown, there is a mountain of evidence to suggest that they are common.

Seemingly contrary to all reason, the energy transaction between psychic vampire and victim is sometimes consensual. Although the psychic vampire is typically the aggressor in consensual interactions, the interaction can be initiated and sustained by either partner. For instance, in codependent relationships, the victim and vampire alike may see vampirism as essential in maintaining the relationship. The victim in such interactions is all too often the enabler who nurtures the vampire relationship.

As already noted, psychic vampirism can be expressed in a modified, disguised form, but with equally detrimental results. Unfortunately, this form of vampirism is often seen on a national scale. As modified vampirism, it typically disregards the rights of other individuals or groups by taking something other than energy away from them. History is replete with instances of oppression, exploitation, and denial of the rights of others, all of which have the fingerprints of vampirism. Even today, this form of vampirism can be seen on a massive scale—ethnic cleansing, institutionalized discrimination, bigotry, ageism, sexism, and racism, all of which reject the dignity and worth of a target individual or group.

Strategy 33

Finger Interlock Procedure

Fortunately, protective procedures are available to prevent a psychic vampire attack, or once it is underway, to promptly extinguish it. The Finger Interlock Procedure is one of the most powerful strategies known for counteracting psychic vampirism and restoring the loss of rejuvenating energy. It combines physical gesture, imagery, and affirmation in a simple step-by-step procedure that not only ends an attack in progress, it energizes the aura and erects a sphere of protective energy, which envelops the aura to temporarily shield it from further assault.

Requiring only seconds to execute, the Finger Interlock Procedure is an all-purpose vampire repellent strategy, which can be used almost anywhere with instant energizing results. The effects of the procedure become immediately visible in the aura, which increases in brightness and intensity, effects that have been illustrated in photographs of the aura taken before and immediately after the procedure. The resultant sphere of bright energy enveloping the aura, which is also called the "halo effect," becomes likewise visible in photographs obtained immediately after the procedure is implemented. (See *Aura Energy for Health, Healing & Balance* for photographs.) Here is the procedure.

Step 1. Finger Interlock Gesture. Begin the procedure by joining the tips of the thumb and middle finger of each hand to form two circles. Next, bring your hands together to form interlocked circles. Hold the finger interlock position for the remainder of the procedure.

Step 2. Energy Protection. Envision a bright sphere of pure energy enveloping your total aura as a shield against any incoming force.

Step 3. Energy Infusion. With the protective sphere in place, sense your aura's innermost core pulsating with power and dispersing vibrant energy throughout your full aura. Let your total being—mind, body, and spirit— become fully infused and revitalized with radiant new energy.

Step 4. Affirmation. Affirm in your own words the empowering effects of the procedure. Examples are: *I am energized and fully enveloped in a protective shield of radiant energy. I am invigorated and fully infused with bright, rejuvenating energy. I am protected, energized, and empowered!*

Step 5. Empowerment Cue. Affirm that by simply forming the interlock gesture, you can at any time instantly reactive the energizing, rejuvenating effects of the procedure.

As already noted, this is an all-purpose procedure with wide-ranging applications. Aside from its primary purpose as a psychic vampire repellent strategy, the procedure can be used to instantly stimulate rejuvenation, manage stress, overcome phobias, improve memory and concentration, break habits, and counteract stage fright, to list but a few. For these applications, Step 4 of the procedure is revised to include additional affirmations relevant to specific goals.

To increase the strategy's rejuvenating capacities, the energy infusion (Step 3) can be expanded to include imagery of the inner fountain of youth being activated and spraying forth bright, rejuvenating energy that infuses the body and bathes it with the glow of youth. The concluding affirmations in Step 4 can be likewise expanded to include additional affirmations relevant to rejuvenation.

Summary

The aura system with its internal core of energy is essential to our pursuit of a younger, longer, better life. The quality of our existence at any moment is largely a function of the aura system. It is a manifestation of the cosmic origin of our existence and a repository of invaluable resources. Fortunately, it is responsive to our intervention. We can use its energies and functions to stimulate the mind, rejuvenate the body, and enliven the spirit. It is unparalleled in its capacity to enrich every facet of our lives.

My book *Aura Energy for Health, Healing & Balance* includes more discussion on the empowering possibilities of the human aura.

CHAPTER 8

Rejuvenation Tools

The use of tangible tools in rejuvenation is based on the concept that certain material objects, when appropriately incorporated into structured procedures, can facilitate the rejuvenation process by either activating it or contributing in some other way to it.

Although tangible objects as rejuvenation tools can be explained from various perspectives, proving objectively their rejuvenation usefulness is a difficult task. In the laboratory setting, two of the many challenges are (1) identifying and controlling the critical variables involved in using material objects as rejuvenation tools, and (2) measuring the short-term and long-term rejuvenation effectiveness of objects and the procedures that use them. Notwithstanding these difficulties, the findings of numerous studies, along with the self-reports of many persons, suggest a very strong relevance of certain tangible objects as rejuvenation tools. Here are some specific ways in which objects are important to rejuvenation.

- The object can assist the imagery process, a critical component of almost all rejuvenation procedures.

- The object, such as a personal jewelry item or even an article of clothing, can possess associative value or symbolic significance that literally stimulates the biological and psychological mechanics of rejuvenation.

- The object, such as a religious symbol, amulet, or charm, can enhance feelings of self-worth and build confidence in one's ability to achieve important goals, including the capacity to master the aging process.

- The object, as a component of the rejuvenation strategy, can provide tangible evidence of one's intent to alter the aging process.

- The object, having been incorporated into an appropriate rejuvenation procedure, can be used as a postprocedure cue to activate or reinforce at any time the rejuvenation process.

- Certain objects seem to be inherently rejuvenating because of their unique makeup. Examples are the quartz crystal, certain gems, and the pyramid. These energized objects can be rejuvenating by their sheer physical presence, but when the object is incorporated into structured procedures, their effectiveness is significantly enhanced.

- Certain objects are useful in rejuvenation because of the expectancy effect; that is, the object's effectiveness as a rejuvenation tool results from our belief in it and our optimistic expectations regarding its use.

- From the interactive perspective, many objects are effective as rejuvenating tools because of our combined psychological, biological, and spiritual responses to the object.

- Certain objects seem to function as channels that connect us to higher sources of unlimited power, to include new dimensions of rejuvenating energy. Other objects seem to directly link consciousness to the vast inner reserves of rejuvenating energy.

- The ideal object functions to activate both inner and outer sources of rejuvenation.

- Flashes of insight and increased feelings of adequacy and personal worth often accompany the use of objects as rejuvenation tools.

The discussion that follows introduces several rejuvenation tools along with strategies that incorporate them. Each strategy recognizes the unique properties of the particular object and its relevance to rejuvenation. It is important to note here that only through practice can you discover the tools and procedures that work best for you individually. Because each tool tends to strengthen or complement the functions of other tools, an ensemble of tools and workable strategies is recommended.

The Quartz Crystal

The quartz crystal is an interesting paradox in that it is at once the oldest and yet newest personal empowerment tool known. It is the oldest in that its empowerment use literally spans centuries. According to legend, ancient Atlantians used the quartz crystal as an indispensable amplifier of cosmic energy. The quartz's anti-aging and attunement properties were widely recognized among Atlantians who applied it throughout the culture. At the demise of Atlantis, again according to legend, the earth was seeded with quartz crystal. So important was this tool that it became firmly etched as an archetype in the consciousness of not only Atlantis but future cultures as well.

Today, the quartz crystal continues to command strong interest as a potential empowerment tool. At the forefront of its wide-ranging applications is an emerging awareness of its age-resistance properties. The contemporary appeal of the crystal is due largely to its receptivity to human programming, whether for rejuvenation or other personal empowerment goals. A given crystal's existing program is easily deleted—a process sometimes erroneously called "cleansing"—and new programming is easily installed, procedures that we will later explain in detail. When appropriately programmed, the crystal can be used to break unwanted habits, master complex motor skills, increase memory, achieve career success, reduce anxiety, and accelerate learning, to list but a few of its wide-ranging applications. Many students have overcome low grades and low self-esteem through procedures that incorporate this important tool.

A crystal for personal use is usually selected from an assortment and then programmed for specific functions. But, incredible as it may seem, the crystal can come to us spontaneously and unexplainably by simply appearing, usually at a conspicuous place in our immediate surroundings as if through some sort of materialization process. Such an amazing appearance signals that the crystal is already preprogrammed to meet a particular personal need which is almost always known intuitively by the recipient.

Even more astounding, a particular crystal with unique identifying features can appear spontaneously again and again in our lives, always for an express purpose or important mission. Over time, the familiar crystal can become an important energizer and collaborator. Upon fulfilling its empowerment role, which may require only a few days, it usually moves on, possibly to help meet the empowerment needs of someone else. At a personal level, a certain clear crystal with a unique signature characteristic—an encased pyramid with rainbow colors—has periodically entered my own life, particularly at times of important transition or decision-making. It first appeared mysteriously at the start of my doctoral studies at the University of Alabama. It appeared in my dorm room and remained with me until I completed the degree, whereupon it vanished as mysteriously as it had appeared. The same crystal later appeared on a laboratory table at Athens State University during a research project designed specifically to develop pain management strategies. As a result of its appearance, we incorporated quartz crystals into the project as potential pain management tools with highly successful results. More recently, the familiar crystal with its telltale features mysteriously appeared on my desk at a time of career transition. In each instance, the crystal's appearance seemed to be empowerment related, and in each instance, it disappeared upon fulfilling its apparent mission.

Along a different line, certain familiar crystals with a history of spontaneous appearances are receptive to deliberate efforts to call them forth whenever they are needed. A highly successful attorney, who had been introduced to crystals as empowerment tools during his undergraduate studies, discovered early in his practice that he could summon a certain familiar crystal through a specially designed meditation strategy in which he communicated with a familiar spirit guide. Invariably, the crystal appeared soon after the meditation. He systematically called forth the crystal during his preparations for important cases or prior to important personal decisions.

Crystals that repeatedly enter our lives and become long-term, interactive collaborators usually possess an array of empowering potentials. As a general rule, they signal a highly positive turn of events in either personal life or career. Usually multiple-programmed, they can empower us to meet demanding situations and help us to achieve important life goals. They can stimulate awareness and generate a sense of balance and well-being. They can provide valuable support and protection as needed.

Crystals that become long-term associates often seem somehow to anticipate our needs. This was illustrated by one of my former students who became a top-level manager in an international communications firm. Notwithstanding his outstanding career achievements, he was unsuccessful in breaking the cigarette habit. Following numerous failed efforts using a variety of strategies designed to break the habit, a striking cluster of amethyst crystals appeared mysteriously on the credenza in his office. Intrigued by its appearance, he stroked the cluster and instantly sensed a personal connection to it. Emboldened by the cluster of crystals, he promptly broke the cigarette habit with complete control. But the work of the mysterious cluster did not stop there. The executive soon discovered that by simply stroking the cluster, he could generate a powerful, positive state of mind. Sensing that the cluster had been multiple pre-programmed, he began using it as a tool for a variety of personal goals, including investment purposes, personal fitness, and rejuvenation. To this day, the cluster of crystals remains at its special place in his office. Its appearance year ago, however, remains a mystery.

Although the effects of crystals that appear spontaneously are typically positive, it is often important to determine the nature of the pre-programming of a particular crystal. Whether the crystal enters our lives spontaneously or as a gift, or when it is selected from an assortment, a simple three-step procedure developed in our laboratory can effectively identify the crystal's pre-programming characteristics. Here is the procedure.

Step 1. Holding. Hold the crystal for a few moments in your cupped palm as you sense its unique physical features, such as shape, weight, warmth, and coolness.

Step 2. Stroking. Stroke the crystal and sense the nature of your interactions with it. Note particularly the responsiveness of the crystal to your touch.

Step 3. Clasping. To determine the crystal's exact mission or program, clasp the crystal between your palms and with your eyes closed, allow impressions and images of the crystal's exact program or mission to emerge in your mind.

This procedure will take a few moments, but you should be patient until the impressions and images appear. If the program or mission of the crystal is compatible with your own goals, you can use the crystal as a personal empowerment tool. Should your interactions with the crystal be incompatible or neutral, you can either discard the crystal or reprogram it as illustrated in Steps 2 and 3 of the Crystal Rejuvenation Procedure that follows.

> *Strategy 34*

Crystal Rejuvenation Procedure

Although crystals can enter our lives spontaneously or as gifts, they are typically selected from either their natural environment or a harvested assortment. Once selected, they can be deliberately programmed for a variety of empowerment goals. The Crystal Rejuvenation Procedure is specifically designed as a guide for selecting, programming, and applying the crystal as a rejuvenation tool.

Step 1. Selecting a Crystal. In selecting an appropriate crystal from an assortment, mentally articulate your rejuvenation goals—arresting aging, becoming revitalized, looking younger, living longer, staying healthy, and so forth—as you pass your hand, palm side down, over the assortment. Notice individual crystals and sense their special energies. Eventually, a certain crystal will "stand out" from the others or seem to "call out" to you. Pick up the crystal and, gently cupping it in your hand, sense your interactions with it. A positive, harmonious interaction confirms the appropriateness of your choice. If you are in doubt, return the crystal to its place in the assortment, and repeat the above process. (Not infrequently, the crystal to be eventually selected is the particular crystal that commanded attention at the beginning of the viewing process.)

Step 2. Clearing the Crystal. To clear the crystal of any previous programming or extraneous energies, simply hold it under cool (not hot) running water for approximately one minute as you stroke it gently with your fingers. You will sense when the clearing process is complete. Place the deprogrammed crystal on a towel and let it air dry.

Step 3. Programming the Crystal. To program the crystal for rejuvenation purposes, hold it in your cupped hand and, with your eyes closed, state your rejuvenation goals. Form mental images of your goals and affirm them as positive expectations rather than some distant, nebulous possibility. For instance, you can picture yourself at your peak of youth with inner biological functions revitalized and all outer signs of aging erased. At this stage, be as imaginative and adventurous as you wish. Give your own energy system permission to interact with the energy system of the crystal. Sense the rejuvenating interaction as it occurs, and invite the crystal to continue to work with you as your partner. In your own words, affirm the reality of the rejuvenation process already initiated through your interaction with the crystal. An affirmation might include: *The energies of youth are now flowing throughout my total being. Mentally, physically, and spiritually, I am renewed. An abundance of anti-aging energy is now at my command. My interaction with the crystal is a fountain of youth that cannot fail.* To complete the programming, address the crystal with the simple message, *Please stay,* which is usually sufficient to save the program.

Step 4. Using the Programmed Crystal. The programmed crystal works best when it is in close proximity to the person. Like programming the crystal, using the crystal for rejuvenation requires physical touch and conscious interaction. During your waking hours, either wearing the crystal as an ornament or carrying it in your pocket or purse is recommended. To unleash its rejuvenation capacities, periodically interact with the crystal by stroking it while envisioning your rejuvenation goals. During sleep, keep the crystal nearby, such as on a bedside table or dresser. Immediately before falling asleep, envision the crystal and sense your connection to it.

A crystal programmed for rejuvenation can be multiple-programmed, but preferably, for related purposes only. Examples are additional programming to ensure healthful sleep, inner attunement, and balance. As a general rule, no more than three programs are recommended for a particular crystal, since too many programs, even when they are related, can interrupt and dilute the crystal's energies.

The Pearl

Only in recent years have we begun to recognize the pearl as an important rejuvenation tool. A 1988 survey, conducted by an experimental parapsychology class at Athens State University, found a strong relationship between exposure to the pearl and longevity. The study interviewed forty women, all over the age of eighty-five. Although the women typically identified the emerald as their preferred gem, it was noted that certain of the women whose complexions were noticeably smooth and wrinkle-free often wore pearls. None of the respondents, however, attributed their youthful features to the pearl. A more recent survey by the author (1996) of a larger population of women, ages seventy-five and over, showed similar results. Admittedly, a limitation of this research was its somewhat subjective nature, along with the possibility that certain uncontrolled variables—social status, wealth, and lifestyle of the women for instance—could explain at least some of the research findings.

Strategy 35

Pearl of Youth

Although the evidence linking the pearl to rejuvenation is limited, we decided to introduce the pearl into a structured rejuvenation procedure called the Pearl of Youth, for use by persons of any age. If simply wearing the pearl is even remotely associated with fewer visible signs of aging, it could be argued that a systematic procedure incorporating the pearl with other known rejuvenation techniques could appreciably influence the underlying aging process. The Pearl of Youth is specifically designed to achieve that goal. Here is the procedure.

Step 1. Selecting the Pearl. A single white pearl is recommended for this procedure. The natural pearl is preferred over the cultured pearl.

Step 2. Finger Roll. As the pearl rests in the palm of either hand, roll the pearl gently between the thumb and fingers of your other hand. Feel the pearl's smoothness and symmetry as you notice the pearl's warm energy interacting with the energies in your fingers.

Step 3. Palm Embrace. Gently hold the pearl between your palms, rolling it slowly. Feel the smooth, warm energies of the pearl interacting with the energies in your hands.

Step 4. Energy Dispersion. With your eyes closed, sense the pearl's soft, smooth energies spreading throughout your body, infusing your total being with radiant new energy. As the pearl continues to rest between your palms, notice again your own energy system interacting with the pearl's gentle, rejuvenating energies. Sense the wondrous serenity accompanying this process.

Step 5. Outer Illumination. With the inner infusion of rejuvenating energy now complete, continue to hold the pearl between your palms as you envision the pearl's energies enveloping your total body with the bright glow of youth. Allow all physical tension, inside and out, to dissolve. Feel the ragged edge of aging slowly vanishing.

Step 6. Pearl Massage. Again, place the pearl in the palm of either hand and gently roll it between the thumb and fingers of your other hand. Notice as before the pearl's energies interacting with the energies of your fingers, then use your fingertips to gently massage your face and neck as the pearl continues to rest in the palm of your other hand. Use a very light touch to smooth away all external signs of aging—wrinkles, puffiness, and sagging muscles. Gently stroke frown lines and crow's feet as you envision them gently vanishing, leaving behind the soft, warm glow of youth. Roll the pearl between your fingers at frequent intervals throughout the massage.

Step 7. Postprocedure Cue. Conclude the procedure by holding the pearl between your palms as you affirm: *By simply stroking the pearl at any time or place, I can instantly generate a powerful, rejuvenating interaction with it.*

You can use the Pearl Massage (Step 6) and the Postprocedure Cue (Step 7) as often as you wish. It is important, however, to periodically repeat the full seven-step procedure. (Note: Because the pearl is soft and easily scratched, it should be kept away from hard objects.)

Following our preliminary studies suggesting a possible efficacy of the pearl as a rejuvenation tool, we designed a study in which ten women and ten men volunteered to practice the Pearl of Youth at two-week intervals over a period of three months. In addition, the participants, whose ages ranged from thirty-eight to fifty-four years, used the Pearl Massage (Step 6) and Postprocedure Cue (Step 7) twice daily (morning and night) over the same experimental period.

At the end of the study, interviews were conducted with each participant to assess the effects of the procedure. The reports of

women participants were consistently positive—they believed
the pearl generated a healthful state of inner balance, while initiating an outer renewal process which was particularly effective
in reducing facial age lines and promoting a soft, smooth com-
plexion. The reports of men participants, some of whom were at
first reluctant to use a procedure they considered "cosmetic,"
were likewise positive. In fact, the self-ratings of men who participated in the study were, on average, greater than the self-ratings of women. One of our subjects, a forty-five-year old male,
used a pearl stickpin, which had belonged to his father, with
highly positive results. Both men and women participants found
the procedure to be effective in removing not only facial age
lines, but also puffiness and sagging facial muscles.

The Pyramid

Another useful rejuvenation tool is a miniature model of the
Great Pyramid. Table models as well as small, hand-held pyramids of a variety of materials—glass, wood, metal, marble,
alabaster, and so forth—have been used effectively as empowerment tools. The key to the pyramid's effectiveness seems to rest,
not in its size or construction material, but in our capacity to
interact with it as a reduced replica in exact proportion to the
Great Pyramid.

Although the sheer physical presence of the pyramid is often
considered empowering, incorporating it into a structured strategy invariably increases its effectiveness. For rejuvenation applications, pyramid strategies focus on not only reversing the
visible effects of aging but also restoring lost mental and physical functions associated with the aging process.

Incredible as it may at first seem, this tool has been
immensely effective in targeting brain activities and restoring
lost mental functions. Using structured pyramid procedures, a
dramatic rewiring of the human brain is not beyond the
intriguing possibilities of this important tool. In the controlled

laboratory setting, improvements in memory, both short- and long-term, along with other cognitive functions have been observed following the introduction of step-by-step procedures using the pyramid. In a particularly interesting study using a rotometer device, our subjects significantly improved their ability to hold a stylus on a moving target after simply holding a small glass pyramid briefly in their hands. In another controlled study, our subjects dramatically improved their ability to recall words that had been presented to them in pairs by simply holding their hands over the pyramid. This simple technique also improved performance in a wide range of athletic activities, including golf, tennis, soccer, and basketball. Along a totally different line, numerous studies have linked the pyramid to the preservation of organic specimen ranging from cut flowers to dead insects, which had been placed inside a hollow pyramid.

$$\boxed{\textit{Strategy 36}}$$

Pyramid of Youth

The Pyramid of Youth is a structured procedure in which a small model of the Great Pyramid is used to promote rejuvenation and longevity. For this procedure, the pyramid can be of any material, but must be small enough to be held in the hand. The Pyramid of Youth is designed to organize our inner rejuvenation mechanisms into a pyramid form that is patterned after the external model. It then links the two pyramids to generate a dynamic rejuvenation event that energizes both mind and body. Here is the procedure that should be conducted in a quiet, comfortable setting.

Step 1. Selecting the Pyramid. Select an appropriate pyramid model that can be conveniently held in the hand. Be careful to select a pyramid replica that is exactly proportional to the Great Pyramid.

Step 2. Pyramid Orientation. Placement of the pyramid, typically on a table, should facilitate a comfortable horizontal or slightly downward gaze. The direction orientation of the pyramid, so long as it rests on its base, does not seem to affect its rejuvenation potential.

Step 3. Pyramid Gazing. Gaze at the pyramid from a comfortable distance as you focus your full attention on it. Following a few moments of relaxed gazing, close your eyes and allow a clear image of the pyramid to emerge. Take plenty of time for the image to form in your mind, preferably as a bright pyramid against a dark background. If you have difficulty forming a mental image of the pyramid, repeat the gazing and imaging sequence until a clear image emerges. Once the image is clearly visible, center your full attention on it.

Step 4. Pyramid Arc of Light. With the pyramid image clearly visible in your mind, envision an arc of bright light connecting the apex of the external pyramid to the apex of your inner pyramid image.

Step 5. Rejuvenation Infusion. With the two pyramids— the one physical and the other mental—linked by the arc of light, envision the outer pyramid pulsating with energy that is, in turn, transferred to the inner pyramid through the arc of bright light. Visualize the inner pyramid, now totally energized, glowing with new power to revitalize every cell and fiber of your body. You can feel the opening of blocked channels and the vibrant flow of new energy. Envision your body now totally enveloped in a rejuvenating glow.

Step 6. Affirmation of Power. Affirm in your own words the rejuvenating effects of the procedure. Examples are: *I am now empowered to defy aging and defeat it. Vibrant new energy is now flowing throughout my total being. I am balanced and attuned to the inner and outer sources of rejuvenation.*

Step 7. Closing Infusion. Place the pyramid in the palm of your hand, and with your other hand palm side down over the pyramid, sense again the powerful infusion of rejuvenating energy.

Step 8. Rejuvenation Cue. As the pyramid continues to rest between your palms, affirm that by holding the pyramid and visualizing the arc connecting it to your inner pyramid, you can instantly unleash abundant youth and health energies to flow throughout your total being.

Although you can reactivate at any time the procedure's effects by using the Rejuvenation Cue (Step 8), the full procedure should be periodically practiced to sustain its powerful effects.

Rejuvenation is only one of the many applications of this procedure. With only minor modifications, it has been used effectively to increase endurance and improve performance in a variety of gym activities. In the clinical setting, the procedure has been used effectively to treat sexual inadequacy, extinguish phobias, and counteract depression and anxiety. In our ongoing studies, there is promising new evidence that the procedure can be used, under appropriate medical supervision, to control pain and accelerate healing. The pyramid, like the quartz crystal, pearl, and certain gems, is an invaluable option in our repertoire of longevity tools.

Using Gems

Our coverage of rejuvenation tangibles would be incomplete without considering the empowering potentials of certain precious gems. Each gem, whether loose or set, seems to emit its own unique energy frequencies; and some gems, like the quartz crystal, appear to function as channels for energy originating external to the gem. But unlike the quartz crystal, each gem seems to be characterized by certain fixed energizing features that appear to be unique to the gem. Although these differential properties can generate a variety of spontaneous energizing effects, they make programming of the gem difficult, and in some instances, as with the diamond, impossible.

Because gems do not readily lend themselves to programming, the selection of gems for rejuvenation purposes is typically based on the recognized inherent properties of the gem. Among the precious gems noted for their rejuvenation potentials are the emerald, amethyst, and sapphire. The emerald is generally recognized for its inherent longevity properties along with its capacity to fortify the immune system. The amethyst is valued primarily for its mental and physical health properties. The sapphire is associated with attunement and social enrichment, including fulfillment of love and affection needs.

Emerald

In repeated surveys, the emerald was found to be the gem of choice among centenarians, many of whom had long recognized its rejuvenation and longevity effects. In an early study by the author concerning the empowering influence of several gems, the emerald was ranked as the number one gem of preference among twenty-seven respondents, age eighty and older. Our study found they were more likely to wear the emerald than any other gem. Although they did not always attribute their longevity to the emerald, they found a certain satisfaction in wearing the gem. As a general rule, the older the respondent the greater their preference for the emerald over other gems. One respondent, age 101, noted that she felt "fully dressed" only when wearing a large emerald pendent, a family heirloom passed down over several generations.

Throughout our surveys, it was found that the emotional connection of our respondents to the emerald, which had often come to them as an heirloom or gift, seemed to enhance its empowering effects. They often provided a detailed history of the gem, which many of them wore daily. One respondent, who often stroked the gem during the interview, viewed it as an important source of mental and spiritual energy. She valued the gem—a gift from her now deceased husband—as a critical link to the discarnate realm. Only rarely did our respondents identify the diamond as their preferred gem, and none of them attributed rejuvenation significance to it.

In view of the strong preference for the emerald by the subjects of our study, and their frequent recognition of the gem's rejuvenating effects, it requires no quantum leap to conclude that the mined emerald, by its design alone, could possibly possess important rejuvenation properties. It would seem plausible that the emerald could emit certain frequencies that interact with our own energy system to slow aging. That possibility, when augmented by a personal belief in the gem's rejuvenating potential, could generate a powerful age-defying process.

Given a wealth of objective evidence of the emerald's rejuvenation properties, we designed two procedures with the emerald as the centerpiece of each procedure. Both procedures—the Emerald Pool and the Emerald Ray—recognize two important sources of rejuvenating energy, one within the self and the other outside the self. Both procedures emphasize the role of the emerald as an external rejuvenation facilitator. They focus on the emerald as a tangible tool that can stimulate our inner capacity to halt aging and restore youthful vigor. At the same time, the procedures do not reject the possible inherent rejuvenation properties of the emerald, but neither procedure depends on these properties alone. Both procedures require the physical presence of the emerald, which can be either loose or set.

Strategy 37

Emerald Pool Strategy

This procedure is structured to promote rejuvenation by flooding the mind and body with youthful energy. It first generates certain positive expectations and then introduces physical touch, mental imagery, self-affirmation, and postprocedure programming, each of which is designed to unleash rejuvenating energy throughout the mind and body. Here is the procedure.

Step 1. Self-Preparation. Find a quiet, comfortable place, and with the emerald resting in your hand, settle back and close your eyes. Clear your mind of all active thought as you become more and more relaxed. As you sense the peaceful serenity and powerful energy enveloping you totally, let yourself become increasingly aware of the supreme power within yourself. Sense the abundant supply of rejuvenating energy poised to be unleashed throughout your total being. Remind yourself of your power to tap the sources of rejuvenation wherever they may exist, and to flood your total being with the healthful energies of youth.

Step 2. Rejuvenating Touch. Gently stroke the emerald, and notice your sense of connection to it. Think of the emerald, not simply as a gem, but as a responsive partner with power to spare. As you continue to stroke the gem, sense its powerful energies flowing into your fingers and interfusing your own energy system.

Step 3. Visualization. With your hands relaxed, visualize the emerald resting in your palm. Sense your attunement to its powerful frequencies. Continue to visualize the emerald with its deep green coloration, and then visualize a still pool of the same coloration. With the image of the pool clear in your mind, imagine yourself diving into it, soaking in its full rejuvenating power. As you remain in the pool, let yourself become renewed and fully infused with bright new energy. Liberate blocked systems, fortify weak organs, and saturate every cell of your body. Stay in the pool until the renewal and infusion process is complete. Finally, visualize stepping from the pool, and bringing forth a sense of total renewal and inner attunement.

Step 4. Self-Affirmation. Affirm in your own words the rejuvenating energy now permeating your total being. Examples: *I am saturated and overflowing with rejuvenating energy. Every fiber of my being is revitalized. Inwardly and outwardly, I am aglow with the radiance of youth.*

Step 5. Postprocedure Programming. The goal of this step is to establish the emerald as a permanent source of rejuvenation. Use the following affirmation to mentally program yourself to initiate on command the emerald's powerful rejuvenation potential: *By stroking the emerald at any time, I will generate a powerful flow of rejuvenating energy. By envisioning the emerald, even when it is not present, I can bathe fully in its rejuvenating glow, thus instantly arresting aging.*

Strategy 38

Emerald Ray Procedure

This procedure introduces imagery of an emerald ray of light connecting the emerald, first to your third-eye region and then to the brain as your body's control center. By establishing a link between the brain and the emerald, the procedure is designed to awaken the brain's renewal potentials and stimulate its rejuvenation mechanisms. As a result, new rejuvenating energies are distributed throughout the physical body. The central and peripheral nervous systems provide the network for infusing the total body with youth and vigor, with the emerald as the key contributing factor. In its capacity to facilitate mental imagery, the emerald seems to spontaneously activate and attune the body's rejuvenation mechanisms. Aging and physical erosion resulting from imbalance and inattunement are spontaneously reversed.

The Emerald Ray Procedure requires the physical presence of the emerald that is held in the hand for the duration of the procedure. Here is the procedure, which requires a comfortable setting free of distractions.

Step 1. Emerald Observation. As you hold the emerald in the palm of your hand, observe its various characteristics, such as size, richness of color, and weight. Stroke the emerald and sense its unique energy frequencies.

Step 2. Emerald Imagery. Close your eyes and envision the emerald. Again, note particularly the gem's physical characteristics, including its energy frequencies.

Step 3. Emerald Ray. As your eyes remain closed, visualize a ray of bright green energy being emitted by the emerald and connecting the stone to the third-eye region of your forehead. Focus your full attention on the bright green ray and note the tingling, energizing sensation at your third-eye region. Think of your third eye as an energy channel and receptive gateway to the brain.

Step 4. Inner Illumination. Allow the bright emerald ray entering your third-eye region to dispel all inner darkness, first dispersing light throughout your brain and then progressively moving downward. Let bright, rejuvenating energy infuse your total body, illuminating it inside and out.

Step 5. Rejuvenation Cue. Affirm in your own words that by simply touching the emerald and then your forehead, while envisioning a ray of bright energy connecting the two, you can fully infuse your body with rejuvenating energy.

Step 5 of this procedure is designed to initiate rejuvenation at any time through a simple gesture and related imagery. This rejuvenation cue can be used almost any place or time. As with other rejuvenation procedures that introduce postprocedure cues, the full five-step procedure should be used periodically to strengthen the cue's effectiveness.

Amethyst

Another gem widely recognized for its rejuvenation properties is the amethyst. As an aura empowerment tool, it can be used to introduce shades of pink or rose into the aura, colors which are associated with healthful mind-body interaction and balance (See my previous book, *Aura Energy for Health, Healing & Balance*). The sheer presence of this gem seems to activate our inner rejuvenation potentials. But as with other gems, when the amethyst is deliberately incorporated into appropriately structured procedures, its rejuvenation potential is significantly expanded.

Strategy 39

Amethyst Amplification Procedure

The Amethyst Amplification Procedure is formulated to expand our rejuvenation resources and direct them toward specific rejuvenation and longevity goals. This holistic, over-the-top procedure not only activates our inner rejuvenation powers, it introduces an outer source of totally new rejuvenation energy. The procedure, which requires the physical presence of the amethyst (either loose or set), integrates inner and outer energy sources, and then balances them to produce an integrated mind-body-spirit state of renewal. The result can be a seismic shift in the aging process.

Step 1. Rejuvenation Touch. While holding the amethyst, note its physical characteristics, paying particular attention to the stone's energy and frequency patterns.

Step 2. Rejuvenation Interaction. As you note the gem's physical features, let yourself respond spontaneously to it. With your eyes closed, sense the emerging interaction, and let it continue to build. Notice especially the attuning effects of the interaction.

Step 3. Rejuvenation Envelope. Hold the gem between your hands in a "praying hands envelope." Sense the gem's balancing effects as the energy interaction builds between your hands. Let the energy generated enter the palms of both hands and spread equally to both sides of your body, finally merging at your solar plexus region.

Step 4. Rejuvenation Amplification. As the energy interaction originating within your hands merges at your solar plexus region, note the burst of bright rejuvenating energy flooding and balancing your total being—mentally, physically, and spiritually. Take a few moments for the process to reach its peak.

Step 5. Rejuvenation Continuum. You are now at your pinnacle of rejuvenation. Your inner fountain of youth is activated and fully energized. Affirm in your own words that you have truly conquered aging and mastered your powers of rejuvenation.

This procedure has been effective for both men and women of various backgrounds and age characteristics. The continuous presence of the amethyst along with periodic use of the Rejuvenation Envelope (Step 3) ensures a continuous state of mental, physical, and spiritual renewal.

Sapphire

Yet another gem considered important for its rejuvenation properties is the sapphire. Traditionally, this gem has long been associated with love, affection, and compassion. Although the mined sapphire exists in numerous colors, the preferred specimen for rejuvenation is the star sapphire with blue tints. When present, it almost always introduces an expansive brightness into the human aura. Among the reported benefits of wearing this gem are increased self-esteem, mental alertness, and self-confidence, as well as mental and physical balance.

In biblical history, the sapphire was a stone of great value. It was the *second* stone in the *second* row of the high priest's breastplate. The number two, according to numerology, signifies balance and antithesis. The gem's placement at *dual* number two positions in the breastplate indicated a healthy balance and a long life for its wearer. Today, the blue sapphire continues to signify longevity and a healthy balance.

Only recently have we begun to explore the rejuvenation properties of the sapphire. Although the studies of this gem have been somewhat subjective and quite varied—they range from laboratory observations to interviews with centenarians—the emerging body of evidence from many sources appears to confirm the gem's valuable rejuvenation properties.

> ## Strategy 40
>
> ### Sapphire of Youth

This procedure is designed to initiate a balanced, internal flow of anti-aging energy. It is a valuable supplement to other rejuvenation procedures in that it can be used almost anytime and anywhere. The simple four-step procedure requires no special conditions other than the presence of the sapphire (either loose or set) and a willingness to use it as a rejuvenation tool.

Step 1. Gazing at the Gem. Begin this procedure by simply gazing at the gem. Note the calming effects of gazing and the emerging state of balance within your energy system.

Step 2. Stroking the Gem. Stroke the gem and note your interaction with it. Pay particular attention to the attuning effects of simply stroking the gem.

Step 3. Holding the Gem. Hold the gem in your cupped hand and sense its energies flowing throughout your total being.

Step 4. Self-Affirmation. To conclude the procedure, affirm in your own words that by simply wearing the sapphire and occasionally stroking it, you can effectively activate its balancing and rejuvenating potentials.

Any of the above procedures using gems as rejuvenation tools can be used in combination with other gems and their related strategies. The concurrent use of various gems for rejuvenation purposes can, in fact, generate a synergistic effect which each gem amplifying the effects of the others.

You may have noticed the absence of the diamond in our discussion of potentially empowering gems. Our studies of the diamond have consistently shown no empowering benefits associated with this popular gem. To the contrary, the physical presence of the diamond has often been associated with numerous negative effects, including fatigue and decreased proficiency in motor performance, particular in activities requiring precision and steadiness of hand. In the laboratory setting, fine motor coordination declined and strength of grip markedly decreased when the diamond was introduced into the experimental situation. Even when the diamond was removed from the experimental situation, the negative residual effects of long-term exposure to the diamond still influenced performance. The large, flawless diamond was found to be particularly detrimental.

Table Tapping

The table may at first seem farfetched as an object with rejuvenation potential. But when we think of table tapping (also known as table tilting) as an interactive phenomenon in which we use a table to "tap into" the discarnate realm and its wealth of empowerment resources, the table assumes considerable importance as a potential rejuvenation tool. Table tapping as applied to rejuvenation holds that the table can become a physical energy channel in which discarnate resources, including rejuvenating energies, can be probed and literally transferred to this physical reality.

Table tapping assumes that the discarnate dimension, rather than a distant reality, is a present though intangible realm with resources that are readily available to us. In addition to rejuvenation and other enrichment energies, discarnate resources include a host of intelligent beings—ministering guides, master teachers, angels, and of course discarnates themselves—all of whom appear responsive to table tapping. They seem, in fact, constantly poised to respond to our probes, and to freely share their invaluable resources.

Like many other self-empowerment strategies, the sheer act of participating in table tapping, independent of stated rejuvenation goals, can be empowering. In a study that introduced table tapping as a voluntary enrichment activity in a retirement living situation, men and women residents who participated in weekly table-tapping session experienced marked improvements in their mood state and medical status. Also, their self-ratings on social satisfaction and personal well-being dramatically increased.

In a study of undergraduate college students, biweekly sessions in table tapping over a six-month period resulted in improved academic performance as well as higher self-rating on such personal traits as self-esteem, optimism, and personal well-being. Furthermore, follow-on assessments revealed important long-term benefits of table tapping.

In addition to these findings, there is considerable evidence that table tapping can directly access certain health and rejuvenating energies of discarnate origin. This has been noted in several studies, including a project conducted at Athens State University where parapsychology students used the procedure to investigate a recurring campus phenomenon. The phenomenon consisted of a green, basketball-sized glow, which appeared sporadically at a second-floor window in Brown Hall, a vacant Greek Revival campus building. Because of the unexplained nature of the glowing sphere, and the possibility that it could be some sort of discarnate manifestation, table tapping was incorporated into a project designed to investigate the phenomenon. Since table tapping appears to literally tap into higher plane energies, it seemed plausible that the procedure could produce the sphere.

In a late-night session, the group of students, equipped with photographic and recording devices, gathered at the site of the recurring phenomenon. Four members of the group were seated around a small table, their hands resting lightly on the tabletop, with the remaining students forming a surrounding circle. Almost immediately, the table tilted to one side and then slowly returned to its original position, whereupon the iridescent green sphere promptly appeared over the table. Temperature probes of the sphere showed readings significantly greater than the surrounding room temperature. Attempts to photograph the sphere, however, were unsuccessful.

As it turned out, the glowing sphere, which was almost always forthcoming in future table tapping sessions, seemed to possess remarkable health and rejuvenation properties. Our early observations found that physical contact with the sphere reduced pain and swelling associated with athletic injury. Later observations found that exposure to the sphere, which became known as "spherical therapy," was highly useful in reducing anxiety and promoting a positive mental state. Without exception, individuals who experienced spherical therapy attested to its enlivening and rejuvenating effects. Unfortunately, the recurring phenomenon ceased when the century-old building was extensively renovated.

Our investigations into the Brown Hall phenomenon are important to our study of rejuvenation because they provide objective evidence of the health and rejuvenation resources existing in other dimensions. Furthermore, they reveal the distinct possibility of accessing those resources and using them to enrich our lives.

Interdimensional Tabling

As a result of our Brown Hall studies, we developed a group procedure designed specifically to probe the discarnate dimension and access its rejuvenation resources through table tapping. The procedure, called Interdimensional Tabling, requires a small table, such as a card table, and at least four participants who are seated around the table with hands resting lightly on the table-top. Interdimensional Tabling is based on the premise that the table, which typically tilts to one side during the procedure, provides an interdimensional tool in which the group's energies interact with those of the discarnate realm.

In its conventional form, table tapping is used basically as a discovery strategy designed to acquire information of discarnate origin. Through its tapping motions, the table can provide "yes" or "no" responses to questions posed by either the participants seated at the table or members of an observing audience. For such applications, one tap of the table on the floor typically signifies a "yes" response with two taps signifying a "no" response. Interdimensional Tabling, on the other hand, goes beyond merely accessing information—it generates a dynamic, two-way interaction with relevance to a wide range of personal concerns, including rejuvenation.

Experiencing the discarnate realm, whatever the nature of the interaction, is almost always rewarding. Interdimensional Tabling is structured primarily to guide the interaction toward a powerful infusion of rejuvenating energy. A secondary benefit of the procedure is the enlightenment that typically accompanies the tabling experience. The procedure includes an optional step (Step 6) expressly designed to further explore the enlightenment resources of the discarnate realm. Here is the procedure.

Step 1. The Setting. Find a quiet setting and set aside approximately one hour for the procedure, which requires at least four participants. A small table, such as a card table (preferably with wooden legs), positioned on a carpeted floor or on the ground, is recommended. Tabling outside by moonlight is thought by some to amplify the rejuvenating effects of the procedure.

Step 2. Participants. Participants can be persons of any age who seek enlightenment and mastery of the aging process. Typically, four volunteer participants are seated at the table. An audience, if present, is usually arranged in a circle with the tabling group at its center.

Step 3. Initial Procedures. The four participants seated at the table initiate the procedure by joining hands while envisioning radiant light of higher cosmic planes enveloping the group. After invoking cosmic guidance in their efforts to interact with the discarnate realm, the participants place their hands—palm sides down—on the table-top and await tilting.

Step 4. Table Levitation. With their hands resting on the table, participants typically experience a mild vibration in the table, followed by actual levitation in which one side of the table rises from the floor. Upon levitating, the table, as a link to higher planes, remains in the tilted position, poised to respond to the group's questions and requests. After expressing their gratitude for the table's receptiveness, participants can invite the table to respond to their questions by tapping on the floor, with one tap signifying "yes" and two taps signifying "no." Either hesitancy or lack of response on the table's part usually suggests the need for clarification or restatement of the question.

Step 5. Rejuvenation. With the table in the tilted position and their hands still resting lightly on the table, participants express, one-by-one, their rejuvenation goals, and request the assistance of higher planes in meeting them. One tap of the table for each request signifies responsiveness of higher planes and full congruency between the individual's goals and available cosmic resources. Upon completing this phase, the table typically remains in the tilted position as rejuvenation energy is channeled to each participant at the table. (At this point, individual members of the surrounding audience can volunteer to participate in the interaction by lightly placing their hands on the tilted table.) Once the energy transfer process is complete, the table typically returns to its original position.

Step 6 (Optional). Enlightenment. Almost invariably, relevant insight accompanies the interdimensional tabling experience. However, participants at this stage of the inter-action often decide to further explore the discarnate realm in an effort to gain further insight. With the energy trans-fer now complete and the table at rest, they first share their enlightenment goals and then invite the table to respond to their questions. As in Step 5, once the interaction is complete, the table will return to its position of rest.

Step 7. Conclusion. Participants customarily conclude the procedure by first expressing their gratitude for the recep-tiveness of the discarnate realm, and then sharing their impressions of the experience.

Individuals of wide-ranging age differences have practiced interdimensional tabling, always with highly positive results. Aside from the procedure's rejuvenation and enlightenment benefits, participants of all ages often experience a dramatic vis-itation of higher plane entities, including the unmistakable pres-ence of advanced spiritual teachers and ministering guides. A student participant who experienced for the first time the dis-tinct presence of his personal spirit guide exclaimed, "It was a peak experience. My life will never be the same." Another par-ticipant, who discovered his spiritual guide during the proce-dure, reported, "It's like I've been reunited with an old and trusted friend."

Summary

Only through practice and experience can we discover the rejuvenation techniques that work best for us individually. It is important to always keep in mind that our rejuvenation needs change over time. Consequently, a workable rejuvenation plan must be both comprehensive and flexible. It must incorporate those strategies that are presently relevant while holding in reserve those options that can be later used as needed.

Strategies using tangible tools are a critical component of any rejuvenation plan. They can range from the use of familiar gems to active participation in group procedures that probe the highest sources of rejuvenating energy. Always, the use of tangibles as rejuvenation tools has many rewards—not least among them are the excitement of new discoveries and the joy of learning new ways to enrich and empower our lives.

CHAPTER 9

Rejuvenation Through Nature

Some of our most valuable empowerment resources are found in our natural surroundings. Examples include our forests, oceans, mountains, streams, plains, and a spectacular array of animal life—all of them manifesting the creative power underlying the existence of all things. When we add to these the whole of the known physical universe, with its billions of galaxies and star systems that invite our probes and interactions, the possibilities are boundless.

Unfortunately, we are often estranged from our natural environment and alienated from its empowering potentials. Yet we have all experienced, in our own way, many wondrous interactions with nature. We have stood in awe before a stalwart tree that scrapes the sky or a desert rock formation sculpted in beauty by wind and sand. We have marveled at the power of a thunderous waterfall crashing relentlessly into a deep cerulean pool, or a magnificent summer rainstorm infusing the earth with bursting rejuvenation. We have been moved by the splendor of a majestic mountain towering steadfastly in quietude, or a serpentine beach stretching and winding its way endlessly along the shimmering sea.

Nature challenges each of us to explore its fathomless array of wonders. By interacting with nature, we can reach new peaks of power and personal insight. From its closest harbinger to its most distant star, nature can connect us to the limitless power that energizes and sustains our very existence. It can enrich our lives with new rejuvenating energy and power. But any serious probe of the empowerment possibilities of nature must begin with ourselves.

We are, like all of our surroundings, a creation of an eternal life force that exists both throughout the cosmos and within ourselves. Each one of us is, at once, both a manifestation and partaker of that force. Without that supreme life force, none of us would exist. Our total being—mentally, physically, and spiritually—is energized by it. All things are possible when we tap into that infinite force. Health, healing, rejuvenation, longevity—they are all within our reach. Even when we finally cross over to the other side, our personal survival as a conscious entity remains a permanent manifestation of that immeasurable force.

In the discussion that follows, we will explore a variety of rejuvenation and longevity resources found in nature. We will develop procedures that focus on a wide range of natural elements and ways we can use them. The procedures are flexible and easily mastered. In fact, a single practice session is usually sufficient, not only to tap into external power sources but to simultaneously unleash the power within ourselves. In most instances, the procedures can be easily altered to fit personal needs, interests, and comfort levels without affecting their overall effectiveness.

The following procedure centers on the tree as a powerful source of rejuvenating energy. When we interact with the tree and its energies, we tap into the planet's strongest life system. It is our planet's oldest and largest living thing. Throughout its lifetime, it never stops growing.

Strategy 42

Tree of Youth

The Tree of Youth is a multifunctional procedure formulated to promote rejuvenating interactions with a selected tree. It is both anti-aging and inspiring in its capacity to balance and attune the human energy system. It actively increases the flow of positive energy by unblocking constricted energy channels. It awakens dormant inner resources while simultaneously accessing higher cosmic sources of rejuvenation. It effectively fortifies our natural immunity against aging by repairing damaged or malfunctioning rejuvenating mechanisms. Simply put, it gives us a rich new lease on life. Here is the procedure.

Step 1. Selecting a Tree. The effectiveness of this procedure rests largely on selecting an appropriate tree. First, it is important to select a tree that appeals to you. Size, age, and type of tree are of only secondary importance. As in selecting a crystal, the tree that commands your attention or seems to beckon you is usually an excellent choice for this procedure. But as a rejuvenation resource, the tree must be more than visually appealing—it must be responsive to your touch. Place your palms against the tree's trunk, and sense its energies. Note the nature of your interaction with the tree and any spontaneous exchange of energies. Sense the compatibility of the two energy systems. Lift your hands a few inches from the tree and note the uninterrupted interaction between your hands and the tree.

Step 2. Naming the Tree. The purpose of this step is to personalize the tree you selected for the procedure by giving it a name. Remind yourself that the tree is an empowerment partner rather than simply a physical object. Think of it as a majestic creation of power and beauty. Then, with your palms again resting upon the tree, close your eyes and assign the tree a name—any name that comes to mind. If you have difficulty naming the tree, use free association by simply saying "tree" and then allowing a name to emerge. (As an aside, many participants of this exercise discovered later on that the name they assigned the tree was the same as that of their ministering guide. This would suggest that personal guides are often spontaneous participants in tree interactions.)

Step 3. Tree Interaction. Although your interaction with the tree actually began with the selection process, it intensifies at this step and finally culminates in a powerful release of rejuvenating energy. As your palms continue to rest lightly against the tree, address it as your rejuvenation partner, calling it by its assigned name. Invite it, in your own words, to interact with you and share its rejuvenating powers. Take a few moments to sense the powerful frequencies of its energies melding with your own energies. Let the tree become a integral part of your own energy system. Sense the powerful transfer of the tree's energy, transforming and rejuvenating your own energy system. Let the tree's rejuvenating energy fully infuse your total being—mentally, physically, and spiritually. Think of the tree as the earth's antenna and your link to the cosmic source of all life. Let yourself become fully attuned to that limitless source of cosmic power.

Step 4. Disengagement. Slowly lift your palms, and while holding them a few inches from the tree, note the continuation of powerful energy infusion. Sense the harmony of the interaction and the wondrous energy resonating throughout your body.

Step 5. Conclusion. Address the tree, and in your own words, express your appreciation for its responsiveness to your rejuvenation needs. Finally, rest your palms again upon the tree and sense its magnificent power. At this point, you may experience a deep and enduring connection to the tree as not only a living system of great power, but a supportive partner in your quest for rejuvenation.

$$\boxed{Strategy\ 43}$$

Nature Walk

All around us, the energies of nature abound, inviting our aware-ness and interaction. The Nature Walk focuses on the many powerful elements found in nature, and our capacity to use them as rejuvenation resources. Nature itself is a rejuvenating, healing force. When we engage its many forms, we generate new possi-bilities for personal growth, rejuvenation, and longevity.

The Nature Walk recognizes the amazing balance of power found in nature. The procedure, which can be used individually or with groups of people, is structured to initiate a rejuvenating interaction with the multiple elements of nature. While engag-ing natural tangibles such as plants, animals, rocks, water, and even soil, the procedure emphasizes nature's spiritual counter-part—the higher creative force that pervades the physical world as well as the cosmos at large.

Although the Nature Walk is primarily a rejuvenation proce-dure, it can be adapted to a variety of other personal goals. It is invariably a source of serenity and balance. New insight and solutions to personal problems often emerge during the walk. Inspiration and a wondrous sense of oneness with nature often accompany the experience. Here is the procedure.

Step 1. The Setting. Select a safe, quiet, and familiar set-ting for your nature walk. Old-growth forests or places with interesting terrain and plant life are particularly ener-gizing. A stream, waterfall, lake, and various rock forma-tions add to the effectiveness of the walk.

Step 2. Preparation. Before starting the walk, take a few moments to relax and reflect on your purposes for the walk. With your eyes closed, take in a few long, deep breaths, exhaling slowly. Let your mind become momen-tarily passive as tranquillity replaces the stresses of everyday life. As you remain relaxed, state your rejuvenation goals as specifically as possibly. Examples include increasing your reserve of age-defying energy, accelerating the rejuvenation process, and even erasing the physical signs of aging. Remind yourself that the possibilities are endless when you free your mind of all self-imposed limitations. When practiced with a partner or group, join hands and affirm together the purposes of the experience.

Step 3. The Walk. Begin your walk by first noticing the rich variety of elements that make up your natural surroundings. Pay particular attention to the myriad of colors, textures, and shapes that, together, form the setting. Listen to the sounds of nature and the messages they bring. Throughout the walk, think of yourself as an integral part of nature rather than separate and apart from it. Sense the creative force that energizes and sustains not only the natural world but your own existence as well. Let your interactions with nature become a gateway to the infinite source of limitless power. Affirm in your own words your interconnection to that invincible source. Take plenty of time for the walk. Pause at frequent intervals, and let your own energy system become synchronized to the energies around you. Sense the rejuvenating power emanating from your surroundings and infusing your total being. Let it envelop you and totally energize the innermost part of your being. Sense the wondrous serenity accompanying the rejuvenation process.

Step 4. Conclusion. Upon completing the walk, pause a few minutes to allow the rejuvenation process to continue unimpeded. Reflect on the walk, and in the group setting, share with the group your personal experiences.

The Nature Walk can be a highly effective component of any comprehensive rejuvenation plan. Although certain anti-aging effects of the Nature Walk are almost always immediately evident, practice increases the procedure's effectiveness. When practiced routinely, it can establish rejuvenation as a continuous, ongoing process of mental and physical renewal.

Strategy 44

Vortex Interactive Strategy

Certain physical settings, because of their location and unique structural designs, are believed to be important intersecting points of powerful energies. At these so-called "power spots," the merging energies from multiple sources can create a synergistic interaction that is sometimes called an *energy vortex*. The vortex typically consists of a powerful energy core that spreads outward in all directions to form an expansive energy field. Like a heat source, the intensity of the energy emitted by the central vortex typically diminishes as it radiates outward.

As a synergistic phenomenon, the vortex is often a powerful cosmic force in which the energies of higher cosmic origin converge with energies of terrestrial origin to produce a highly charged field of finely tuned frequencies. When we enter the vortex, we become spontaneously energized participants in that synergistic interaction. We can then deliberately engage the vortex, tap into its powerful energies, and direct them toward specific empowerment goals, to include mental and physical rejuvenation.

Typically a stationary phenomenon, the energy vortex is often found in places known for their natural beauty, including deserts, plains, mountainous regions, forests, and river intersections. Native Americans were particularly aware of energy vortexes, and they often selected them for their settlements and burial grounds.

Certain energy vortexes are believed to be important gateways to higher cosmic dimensions. Upon entering the gateway vortex, we become, often instantaneously, energized and attuned. By lingering in the gateway vortex, we can often experience the presence of higher plane entities, including ministering teachers and guides. The results can be profound enlightenment and expanded awareness of other dimensions.

Mountain peaks are among the common vortex sites with strong rejuvenation potential. Throughout recorded history, mountains, which make up about a fifth of the land surface of the world, have intrigued civilizations past and present. Although mountains presented challenges to travel and communication, they were valued for their usefulness and beauty. Ancient civilizations were struck in awe of them, often viewing their highest peaks as the habitation of gods. The ancient Incas considered mountains sacred, the higher the mountain the greater its spiritual significance. Other examples include Mount Fuji, which remains sacred to many Japanese, and Mount Sinai from which, according to biblical accounts, Moses was given the Ten Commandments. It was on a mountain that Noah's ark came to rest following the great flood. It was on a mountain that Jesus prayed prior to his crucifixion, and it was on a mountain that he was crucified. The vortex nature of mountains could help explain its prominent role in the history of civilization as well as its contemporary appeal. Mountain climbing, for instance, could be explained as a vortex attraction. The experience is often described by climbers as inspiring and intensely exhilarating.

Other common energy vortex locations are old-growth forests and the interior regions of island groups formed by submarine mountains, such as the West Indies. In some instances, the vortex energies interact with gravity to generate a near weightless situation. In the northern region of Alabama, a certain mountainous road crosses an apparent vortex with energies so powerful that they literally stall automobiles traveling at low speeds. Also in northern Alabama, a small valley area is known for its constant easterly breeze, a phenomenon that meteorologists have described as "mystifying." On the Atlantic coast of

Florida, a certain stretch of beach has a vortex that is believed to forcibly shift the direction of the sea breeze. Rather than incoming from the sea, the breeze in the vortex is typically outgoing. Other examples of possible energy vortexes are the Bermuda Triangle and certain mountainous regions of Peru.

It is probable that powerful energy vortexes exist throughout the physical universe. For instance, the moon seems to possess characteristics that could be explained as vortex energies. Supportive of that possibility are the numerous phenomena, including certain changes in human behavior, which are often associated with moon phases. The fact that the lunar orb has often been romanticized in poetry and song, incorporated in rituals, and even worshipped adds further credence to the possibility of important lunar vortex influences. It is also plausible that the arrangement of planets and other heavenly bodies in their relationship to the earth could generate powerful but at times transient vortex conditions. Although that influence could dramatically affect our individual behavior, many permanent earth vortexes seem to be influenced only mildly, if at all, by normal variations in extraterrestrial conditions.

It is conceivable that certain geographical regions, including those remote areas found in Asia, which are known for the longevity of their inhabitants, could be vortexes with highly positive rejuvenating energies. Not infrequently, residents of these regions surpass a hundred years in age, with incredibly excellent health.

Unfortunately, not all vortex energies are positive. Energies from multiple sources can converge in ways that result in a highly negative force. Although negative vortex energies are often exaggerated, exposure to such conditions, particularly if prolonged, can be harmful to both mind and body. Examples are certain architectural structures including bridges, houses, and industrial and business facilities, which are associated with recurring illness, failure, and even death. Our health and success may depend, at least in part, on the vortex energies of the home and workplace. While the rearrangement of furnishings can, to some degree, offset the negative effects of the vortex, they seldom can totally eliminate them. Similarly, metaphysical and religious efforts, including various "cleansing" and "exorcising" rituals, have been only marginally effective in counteracting the negative vortex.

Although typically a natural phenomenon, the positive energy vortex can be deliberately generated, a phenomenon illustrated by certain spectacular engineering feats such as the Great Pyramid and Stonehenge. Native Americans, who were, as already noted, sensitive to the energy vortex, may have deliberately generated certain vortexes through their ceremonial rites. Interestingly, the herbal garden is often a highly energized vortex with both healing and rejuvenating properties, particularly when the plants are arranged in circles within circles. By meditating in the center of the garden's innermost circle, we can tap into the collective healing and rejuvenating energies the vortex attracts, as well as those generated by its living plants.

The Vortex Interactive Strategy is structured to initiate a rejuvenating vortex interaction and to target positive vortex energies to designated goals. It views the vortex as both a generator and repository of energy. The procedure can be used to maximize the effects of an existing natural vortex, or to erect a totally new energy vortex system, which can be relatively permanent. When used for the home, office, or other workplace, the procedure can generate conditions that attract positive cosmic energies of the highest level. The procedure can be implemented as either an individual or group exercise. Here is the procedure.

Step 1. The Setting. The setting for this procedure can be an existing energy vortex or wherever a new vortex is to be erected.

Step 2. Vortex Centering. While situated in the interior region of either the existing vortex or the proposed new vortex, envision the vortex as a cone-like formation with the circular base forming the earth boundary and the peak of the cone serving as a receiver of energy from the highest cosmic realm. Affirm your intent to either maximize the power of the existing vortex or to generate a totally new vortex. Envision the cone of the vortex as pointing to the bright energizing core of the cosmos.

Step 3. Vortex Moorings. Establish vortex moorings through the *perimeter walk,* in which you either step-off a circle around the existing or proposed vortex's inner region; or in the group situation, form a circle around the vortex's inner region with members of the group either holding hands or spaced at approximate equal distances. Establishing vortex moorings inside the existing or proposed vortex seems to concentrate the power of the larger vortex within the newly designated interior region.

Step 4. Vortex Interaction. Return to the center of the existing or proposed vortex and with your eyes closed, envision again the vortex as a cone-like formation with its central core focused on the cosmic core of pure energy. Sense the building energy within the vortex, and allow yourself to become increasingly infused with it. Let pure cosmic energy fully permeate your total being—mentally, physically, and spiritually. Sense the renewal of your own energy system as it interacts with your cosmic origins. You are now attuned completely, totally balanced and imbued with new vitality. Your entire existence is enriched by the new surge of power within.

Step 5. Goal Statement. State your empowerment goals, which can include an extensive range of personal objectives, including mental and physical rejuvenation. Envision each goal as clearly as possible, and affirm your power to achieve it.

Step 6. Energy Diffusion. From your position within the existing or proposed vortex, turn your hands outward and move them slowly from side-to-side to distribute new energy evenly throughout the total vortex.

Step 7. Conclusion. Conclude the procedure with expressions of gratitude for the abundant energy of the highest level.

Individuals, couples, and groups can use this procedure to improve their quality of life. While rejuvenation is among its benefits, its energizing and enrichment effects are unlimited. In couples counseling, it has been used with great success as an assigned home exercise to strengthen relationships and solve marital problems, including financial. In the organizational setting, it can be used to increase commitment to organizational goals and promote positive group interactions. Every home and work environment can be energized and enriched through this simple procedure.

Strategy 45

Inner Vortex Strategy

Typically, the energy vortex is considered an environmental phenomenon. Its origin can be either natural or deliberately contrived. In both forms, the energy vortex is receptive to our intervention. As already noted, we can interact with the vortex and effectively activate its empowerment potentials, including rejuvenation.

Just as the external energy vortex can be deliberately generated through structured procedures, such as the above Vortex Interactive Strategy; we can establish a vortex within the self that can become our link to the highest cosmic source of pure energy. The Inner Vortex Strategy is designed to achieve that goal. Here is the procedure.

Step 1. Goal Statement. State your intent to establish an energy vortex within yourself. Specify the empowerment functions of the vortex, such as rejuvenation and longevity or any other personal empowerment goal.

Step 2. Vortex Cone. While lying down and with your eyes closed, envision your solar plexus region as an abundant repository of bright energy. Using either hand, initiate circular clockwise motions a few inches from your body at your solar plexus region. Envision energy from your solar plexus becoming activated to spin clockwise, thus establishing a base for the vortex. Continue the clockwise motions using your hand's circular motions to form a spiraling cone of luminous energy rising from your body, with the solar plexus constituting the vortex's energizing base.

Step 3. Cosmic Infusion. With the spiraling cone of energy rising above your solar plexus, envision a bright beam of radiant energy connecting the apex of the vortex cone to the distant cosmic core of pure energy. Sense powerful energy infusing the vortex and then spreading throughout your body. Note the balancing, rejuvenating effect of the experience.

Step 4. Concluding Affirmation. Conclude the procedure with positive self-affirmations related to your goals as stated in Step 1. Examples are: *I am at my peak of personal power. The energies of my being are attuned to the cosmic source of my existence. I am at one with the cosmos.*

Human-Animal Interactions

The animal kingdom (that is, all nonhumans) is yet another vast repository of important rejuvenating potential. By living with animals and interacting with them as their guardians—not owners—we can enrich our lives with exciting new growth and joy. But critical to that interaction are our appreciation of animals and our awareness of their preeminent place in the larger cosmic scheme. Here are some important considerations that together provide the foundation for rewarding interactions with animals.

- They are beings of dignity and worth.

- They deserve our respect and protection.

- As friends rather than property, they teach us many important lessons—devotion, trust, courage, loyalty, affection, and resilience.

- They often bring peace, comfort, and joy into our lives.

- They can help meet our needs for renewal, playfulness, relaxation, and acceptance.

Animals manifest nature's energy in one of its most basic yet purest form. They are enveloped in an aura of energy that is luminous and free of discoloration and imbalance. By living and interacting with them, we experience a wondrous renewal of our energy system as well as the sheer pleasure of the interaction.

Summary

Nowhere are the possibilities for rejuvenation and abundant living more evident than in our natural surroundings. Nature provides more than the essential conditions for our physical survival, it offers a vast array of resources that can enrich our lives. From the smallest particle of matter to the most distant star system, nature manifests the creative cosmic force underlying our very existence. Through our interactions with nature, we come to know that life force, and even more importantly, we become as one with it. That oneness is, perhaps, the most powerful rejuvenating force of all.

Chapter 10

A Seven-Day Rejuvenation Plan

As we enter a new millennium, we turn a new corner of opportunity. We now know that most of the "limitations of old age" are stereotypical rather than real. For the most part, things that were once seen as beyond our control can now be modified or reversed. Furthermore, we can take pre-emptive action to eliminate the need for corrective action later on. Thanks to a new rejuvenation technology that recognizes the supreme power of the mind and spirit, senescence is neither inevitable nor irremediable. We can master strategies that trigger rejuvenation and prolong life while enjoying all-around good health. Rather than self-destructing, we can literally create a new design for living younger, longer, and better.

This chapter presents a series of strategies drawn from previous chapters and organized into a seven-day plan designed to counteract aging and initiate an upward spiral of rejuvenation. The plan for each day specifies goals and relevant strategies for achieving them. The plan begins with certain basics, such as ways to manage negative stress, and then progresses to more complex procedures that include interacting with other dimensions. The plan culminates in procedures that link the mind, body, and spirit to the highest cosmic source of rejuvenation.

The inner and outer sources of rejuvenation are now at your command. Through this plan, you can take swift, decisive action to stimulate your inner fountain of youth while accessing the supreme cosmic fountain of limitless possibilities.

Day One

Goal: To eliminate negative stress and replace it with abundant rejuvenating energy.

Negative stress is a dangerous serpent in the garden of rejuvenation. It accelerates aging and shortens our lives. Day one introduces two procedures designed to promote physical relaxation, eliminate negative stress, and help repair its wear and tear effects. The Toe-lift Technique uses a simple physical gesture to induce a tranquil, relaxed mental state and flood the body with rejuvenating energy. The Control Center Strategy intervenes into brain activity to induce relaxation, slow the aging process, and reverse the biological effects of aging.

Toe-Lift Technique

Step 1. Preliminaries. In a comfortable, quiet setting, settle back and clear your mind of all active thought. Slow your breathing, and let all your cares gently roll away, like boulders rolling down a hill and into the sea.

Step 2. Toe Lift. Slowly raise your toes, and hold them in the raised position. If you are wearing shoes, press your toes gently against the top of your shoes. Hold the position as you sense tension building in your muscles, first in your feet and lower legs, then into your thighs, and finally throughout your body. Continue to hold the toe-lift position until the tension reaches its peak, typically within a minute or two.

Step 3. Relaxation. With the tension now at its peak, very slowly relax your toes, and allow them to finally reach their original position. With your toes now at rest, let the relaxation erase all tension by spreading gently upward, first into your ankles and lower legs, then slowly rising to infuse your total body. Take plenty of time for your body to become totally relaxed, from your feet to your forehead.

Step 4. Rejuvenating Mist. With your body now in a state of deep relaxation, envision a mist of bright, rejuvenating energy gathering around your feet and gently rising to envelop your total body. Sense your body absorbing rejuvenation from the tips of your toes to the top of your head.

Step 5. Glow of Youth. Breathe in the mist of bright rejuvenating energy, taking it deep into your lungs. Hold your breath for a moment, and allow the bright energies of youth to spread throughout your body, saturating joints, fibers, tendons, organs, and systems with radiant rejuvenating energy. Sense youthful vitality permeating every cell of your body. Envision your body enveloped in the glow of youth.

Step 6. Targeting Rejuvenation. Select specific physical signs of aging and mentally bathe each one with bright anti-aging energy. Envision rejuvenation as concentrated laser-like beams gently erasing the physical signs of aging and energizing your body's every function.

Step 7. Affirmation. As you remain deeply relaxed, affirm: *I am free of negative stress and fully infused with positive energy. Rejuvenation is now flowing throughout my total body.*

Step 8. Toe-Lift Cue. Conclude with the following rejuvenation cue: *I am empowered to eliminate negative stress and replace it with rejuvenation at any moment by simply raising my toes and affirming: I am relaxed and totally infused with the positive energies of youth.*

You can use the Toe-lift Cue (Step 8) almost anywhere and under almost any condition to infuse the mind and body with positive energy.

Control Center Strategy

Step 1. Relaxation. Find a quiet, comfortable place, settle back, and focus your attention briefly on your breathing. Take in a few deep breaths, holding each breath for a few moments before slowly exhaling. Think of yourself as breathing in positive energy and exhaling negative energy. With your eyes closed, develop a relaxed, rhythmic breathing pattern as you become more and more relaxed. Affirm: *I am calm, relaxed, and at complete peace with myself and the universe.*

Step 2. Brain Imagery. Center your thoughts on the dark, interior region of your brain. Envision your conscious presence in the brain as a light-form illuminating the innermost regions and pathways of your brain.

Step 3. Brain Rejuvenation. Probe your brain's darkest central regions as you emit light from your conscious presence there. Slowly expel the darkness until your brain is aglow with bright energy. Allow the light of your presence to fully permeate your brain—energizing, rejuvenating, and revitalizing its activities. Your brain is now radiating bright, powerful energy.

Step 4. Inner Rejuvenation. From your control position at the brain's central region, use imagery to disperse positive energy in bright light-form, first into your solar plexus region and from there, throughout your total body, driving away all the dark residue of negative stress until you are fully infused with light and positive energy. Bathe each physical organ with the light of health and rejuvenation. Take plenty of time to energize every physical organ and system with vitality and healing energy. Give stress-damaged and dysfunctional organs permission to heal and function normally.

Step 5. Outer Rejuvenation. While maintaining your control position in the brain, expand the energy emanating from your solar plexus until your physical body is enveloped fully in a powerful, expansive field of bright, rejuvenating energy. Give all outward manifestations of aging permission to slowly dissolve.

Step 6. Balance and Harmony. Envision your brain, solar plexus, and surrounding energy field interacting and working together in total harmony, all under the direction of your conscious mind.

Step 7. Rejuvenation Cue. As you envision yourself enveloped in bright energy, bring your fingers to your temples as a gesture to signify the infusion of positive, rejuvenating energy throughout your total being. Affirm in your own words your power to instantly reduce stress and activate rejuvenation at any time by simply closing your eyes and touching your temples as you envision yourself enveloped in powerful, bright energy.

Once you master this procedure, you can effectively apply the Rejuvenation Cue (Step 7) as often as needed.

Day Two

Goal: To promote physical and mental renewal through sleep and awakening strategies.

Day two of our plan introduces two strategies that capitalize on the rejuvenation potential of sleep. The Sleep Anti-aging Strategy emphasizes both physical and mental renewal. Improvements in both mood state and memory almost always accompany the regular use of this procedure.

The second procedure, Awakening Rejuvenation, accesses our inner rejuvenation resources by capturing the few moments of somewhat semiconsciousness characterizing the natural awakening state. It requires either spontaneous awakening or gradual awakening, such as to soft music or other pleasing sounds. Both procedures should be practiced daily for the remainder of the seven-day plan.

Sleep Anti-aging Strategy

Step 1. Presleep Conditioning. Prior to falling asleep, reflect on your immediate and long-term rejuvenation goals, both physical and mental. State them clearly in your mind, and think of them as not only goals but as also future realities. Assign to each goal a bright, crystalline form, with each luminous form representing a biological system or mental function to be revitalized and renewed. For instance, a cube can represent healthy cell reproduction, a pyramid can represent mental alertness, and a sphere can represent a strong immune system. Envision the forms as small enough to hold in the hand.

Step 2. Imagery. With your eyes closed, envision your subconscious mind as a clear pool of abundant rejuvenating energy. Picture yourself at the edge of the pool with the crystalline forms in your hands. Imagine yourself tossing the forms, one by one, into the pool. As each form sinks deeper and deeper, remind yourself that the fluid energy enveloping each form is saturating the mental or physical function it represents. Sense the flow of rejuvenating energy permeating your body. Continue to envision the clear pool with its crystalline forms until sleep ensues, typically within a few minutes.

Step 3. Postsleep Conditioning. Upon awakening, review your rejuvenation goals and affirm your power to achieve them. Envision again the clear pool with its crystalline forms. As you hold the image clearly in your mind, erect a triangle by first joining the tips of your thumbs to form its base and then joining the tips of your index fingers to form its top. Affirm that by simply forming the so-called Triangle of Power as you envision the pool with its forms, you can instantly activate at any time the flow of rejuvenating energy throughout your body.

This procedure can be easily modified to include relevant imagery and affirmations related to other empowerment goals. The Triangle of Power (Step 3) can be used as often as needed to reinforce the effects of the full procedure.

Awakening Rejuvenation

Step 1. Body Imagery. As you begin to spontaneously awaken from sleep, form an image of your physical body as you continue to rest comfortably with eyes remaining closed.

Step 2. Facial Renewal. Imagine yourself with a pencil eraser in hand, gently erasing the visible signs of aging, such as lines around your eyes or mouth. To restore youthful muscle tone, visualizing yourself placing a comfortable mask of youth over your face. Sense the firmness in the muscles as your face conforms to the mask.

Step 3. Full-Body Renewal. Envision yourself slipping into a form-fitting rejuvenation garment. Sense the gentle shaping of your body to the youthful proportions of the garment.

Step 4. Aura of Youth. Envision the mask and garment slowly fading, taking with them the signs of aging and leaving behind only the radiance of youth. Sense the glowing aura of youth enveloping your body.

Step 5. Inner Renewal. Envision the central region of your body radiating a youthful glow that saturates your total being, inside and out. Allow rejuvenating energy to infuse every organ and system of your body.

Step 6. Concluding Affirmation. Affirm: *Throughout this day, I will be at my peak of power and youthful vitality. The* *energies of youth will flow continuously throughout my total being.*

Like the Sleep Anti-aging Strategy, Awakening Rejuvenation is a flexible procedure which you can adapt as needed to meet highly specific rejuvenation goals as well as a wide range of health and fitness needs.

Day Three

Goal: To tap the highest cosmic source of rejuvenation and to discover higher plane entities.

Day three is a critical point in our seven-day plan. It introduces three strategies designed to access the rejuvenating power of the higher cosmos. The first strategy, Cosmic Infusion Procedure, views cosmic energy as white light which can be readily accessed and absorbed throughout the body to infuse it with rejuvenation and balance. The second strategy, Cosmic Interaction Strategy, is specifically structured to reveal higher plane entities—particularly rejuvenation specialists—who can help us master the aging process by opening new growth channels and increasing the inner flow of rejuvenating energy. The third strategy, Higher Plane Rejuvenation, accesses the green cosmic plane that appears to be situated near the bright center of the cosmos. That plane, which is directly energized by the cosmic core, transforms pure life-force energy into a rejuvenating form, which is responsive to human interaction. By interacting with the green plane, we can revitalize and renew the physical body.

Cosmic Infusion Procedure

Step 1. Goal Statement. In a quiet, comfortable setting, affirm your goal of achieving a state of full cosmic infusion of rejuvenating energy—mentally, physically, and spiritually. State your rejuvenation objectives as specifically as possible.

Examples include slowing the aging process, revitalizing the mind and body, activating anti-aging processes, erasing the physical signs of aging, strengthening and enhancing specific brain functions, and restoring mental and physical powers, to mention but a few of the possibilities.

Step 2. Relaxation. As you remain quiet and comfortable, settle back and take in several deep breaths, pausing briefly between breaths. Continue to focus on your breathing until you develop a comfortable, rhythmic breathing pattern. Think of each breath as "taking in" relaxation and "letting go" tension. Let your muscles become loose and limp as you release all physical tension, replacing it with deep relaxation.

Step 3. Energy Infusion. Turn your palms upward and think of your hands as your body's antennae to the cosmos. Envision the discarnate realm as a dimension of pure white light. Let bright beams of cosmic light enter your palms and then spread throughout your total body, balancing and energizing your total being. Sense the energy soaking deep into every fiber, muscle, and joint, infusing every vital organ and system with rejuvenation. (At this point, you may experience warm, tingling energy, first in your palms and then deep within your body.) Target rejuvenating energy to specific body areas. Allow plenty of time for the infusion event to reach its peak.

Step 4. Conclusion. Affirm your power to tap at will the resources of higher planes, and to use them to achieve your rejuvenation goals. This procedure can be practiced at any time and as often as preferred.

Cosmic Interaction Strategy

Step 1. Letting Go. Settle back and, with your eyes closed, clear your mind of all active thought. Then, as you remain relaxed, allow new thoughts and images to slowly flow in and out of your mind. Make no effort to arrest these thoughts and images as you experience the calming effects of simply "letting go." Allow this free-flowing process to continue until smooth tranquillity replaces the ragged edges of stress.

Step 2. Childhood Reverie. As you remain in a passive, relaxed state, allow images of your childhood to flow in and out of your mind. Let the images freely come and go until a particularly pleasant image of an early childhood event enters your mind. Focus on the event for a few moments, then give yourself permission to drift back in time to re-experience it exactly as it occurred. Allow plenty of time for you to become completely absorbed in the unfolding event. In that state of reverie, sense the wonderment of your childhood and the freedom from all your accumulated cares.

Step 3. Cosmic Infusion. Now free of your adult baggage, let yourself sense anew the inner attunement and oneness with the cosmic source of your existence. As you linger in the reverie state, note your feelings of wondrous congruency with the cosmos. Sense the nurturing resources of the higher cosmos, and remind yourself that they are now available to you. Expand your awareness to include the presence of ministering guides and teachers along with caring angels and other spiritual helpers, some of whom will probably seem familiar to you. Take plenty of time to renew your awareness and appreciation of them. Remind yourself that they are your present helpers. You can invite them to guide your pursuit of rejuvenation as well as other important goals in your life. Sense the rejuvenating power of your interactions with them as the glow of youth envelops your body. Let the interaction and energizing process continue until your are fully infused with rejuvenating cosmic energy.

Step 4. Into the Present. The cosmic infusion processes now complete, shift your attention to the present and your immediate surroundings. Remind yourself that the supreme cosmic forces that energized your existence from the beginning are constantly present to enrich your life with all the abundant resources of the cosmos.

Step 5. Conclusion. Affirm your ability to reactivate the effects of this procedure at any time by simply reflecting on the early childhood experience and opening your mind to the wondrous presence of higher plane entities. Almost everyone who practices this procedure experiences a sense of wonderment at their rediscovery of "forgotten" higher plane acquaintances.

Higher Plane Rejuvenation

Step 1. Solar Plexus Centering. Close your eyes and center your full attention on your central body region. Envision that inner region filled with light which radiates throughout your body. Imagine the innermost part of your body—deep within your chest and abdomen—bathed with radiant light. Sense the release of tension as the light expands to illuminate your total body—organs, systems, joints, and muscles. Absorb the bright light deeper and deeper into every cell of your body.

Step 2. Outer Illumination. Let the radiance permeating your total body slowly expand, enveloping your full body in an aura of bright energy. Envision the aura of energy expanding and radiating outward.

Step 3. Cosmic Core Imagery. Envision the distant core of the cosmos as a radiating dimension of light in its purest form. Remind yourself that the cosmic energy core is the cradle of creation and the energizing source that sustains your existence.

Step 4. The Green Plane. Notice an expansive, iridescent green plane reaching outward from the shining cosmic core and radiating bright beams of energy in all directions throughout the universe.

Step 5. Energy Infusion. Turn the palms of your hands upward toward the green plane, and let its radiating beams of bright energy soak into your hands. Think of your hands as powerful receptors of cosmic energy. Sense the infusion of energy spreading from your hands to your solar plexus, and from there, throughout your body.

Step 6. Rejuvenation. Take a mental journey through your body by first scanning your body, beginning with your upper body region. As you progressively scan your body downward, bathe every cell and fiber with bright radiant energy. Target any problem area—a weak organ, dysfunctional system, or area of pain—and saturate it with bright, rejuvenating energy. Notice the warm, tingling, anti-aging energies flowing throughout your body.

Step 7. Balance. Upon completing the body scan, bring your hands together in a praying hands position to balance the infusion process and fully attune your mind, body, and spirit to the cosmic source of your existence. Affirm in your own words the rejuvenating results of the procedure.

Step 8. Reactivation. The rejuvenating effects of this procedure can be reactivated at any time through the following three steps, which require only a few seconds. (1) Turn your palms upward as you envision radiant green energy infusing your total body with rejuvenation; (2) use the praying-hands gesture to balance the new infusion of energy; and (3) affirm the powerful rejuvenating effects of the strategy.

Day Four

Goal: Day four's goal is twofold; first, to generate a state of general empowerment and renewal, and second, to energize and balance your inner fountain of youth with the outer cosmic fountain of unlimited rejuvenation.

Day four introduces two important strategies, both of which use astral travel. The first, Destination Travel, uses out-of-body procedures to promote a state of general empowerment. It generates a positive, optimistic state of mind, a condition that is critical to rejuvenation. The rejuvenation results seem to be greatest when the destination relates to youth. The second strategy for day four, the Cosmic Fountain of Youth, guides astral travel to the fountain where the astral body is bathed in a sparkling spray of rejuvenating energy. This procedure energizes and balances the inner fountain of youth with the outer cosmic fountain of unlimited rejuvenation.

Destination Travel

Step 1. Preliminaries. Settle back, take in a few deep breaths, and develop a comfortable, effortless breathing pattern. In your own words, invoke astral guidance while envisioning yourself enveloped in bright astral light.

Step 2. Induction. Clear your mind of all active thought, and with your eyes closed, focus only on your breathing for a few moments. Shift your attention to the innermost part of yourself, and envision that part as a bright light-form. Let that glowing form gently rise above your body, taking on a light-form of your physical body, and transporting with it your conscious awareness. Take plenty of time for this process to unfold. Once the light-form embodying consciousness is suspended over your physical body, observe your body at rest below for a few moments. Stay with that external locus of awareness until you've firmly established a full sense of being out of your physical body. Remind yourself that you are secure and protected by all the positive forces of the universe.

Step 3. Destination Control. As you remain out-of-body, select a favorite place—perhaps a safe retreat or a carefree setting from childhood with its rich memories—and give yourself permission to go there. Hold the clear image of your destination firmly in your mind until your experience the full reality of being there. (Note: This step is based on the concept that, in the out-of-body state, imagery combined with intent generates the essential vehicle for travel to selected destinations, whether on this earth plane or at some distant point in the cosmos.)

Step 4. Renewal. Having reached your destination, view your surroundings, and notice your sense of pleasure and personal fulfillment. Breathe in the wondrous energies enveloping you. Let the infusion of energy continue until you are totally energized and at your peak of full renewal.

Step 5. Goal Attainment. Envision your personal goals and affirm them in your own words as realities, as either works in progress or already fulfilled. For rejuvenation, first envision yourself at your youthful prime, and then affirm your capacity to physically manifest that vision. For other goals, regardless of how varied they may be, envision them as realities—present or future—and affirm your power to experience them.

Step 6. The Return. To return to your physical body, turn your attention again to your body at rest, and give yourself permission to re-unite with it. Upon re-entering your body, notice your physical sensations—breathing, heartbeat, body weight, and so forth—as signals of your return.

Step 7. Self-Empowerment Affirmations. With your astral and biological bodies now reunited, briefly review your out-of-body experience and in your own words, affirm its empowering effects. Examples are: *Bright, rejuvenating energy is now flowing throughout my total being. I am infused with youthful vitality. I am at my peak—mentally, physically, and spiritually. I am fully empowered to achieve my personal goals of* (state goals).

Step 8. Postprocedure Cue. Conclude the procedure with the affirmation that simply envisioning the out-of-body destination selected for this procedure, and yourself interacting with it, is sufficient to instantly reactivate the procedure's empowerment effects.

Cosmic Fountain of Youth

Step 1. Induction. Induce the out-of-body state by following Steps 1 and 2 of the Destination Travel as previously presented.

Step 2. Cosmic Travel. As you remain out of body, view the cosmos with its many planes, pathways, and other forms. Search the cosmos until you discover a bright green energy plane. Give yourself permission to engage the plane, and upon entering it, let yourself be drawn to its innermost region where you will discover a sparkling fountain with its arching spray of bright energy. Allow plenty of time for you to engage the plane and its innermost region. Once comfortably in the presence of the plane's fountain, enter the fountain's spray and let its streams of invigorating energy bathe your astral body. Sense rejuvenating energy rising from your inner fountain of youth, then merging with the outer fountain's spray of rejuvenating energy. Let the inner and outer merging of energy continue until your inner fountain becomes totally energized, balanced, and attuned to the outer cosmic fountain of abundant energy.

Step 3. The Return. With your inner fountain now fully functional and completely energized, step from the fountain and turn your attention to your physical body at rest. Give yourself permission to return to your physical body and reunite with it. Upon merging with your physical body, sense the powerful infusion of cosmic energy rejuvenating every fiber, muscle, joint, and tendon of your body. Sense the wear-and-tear effects of stress and aging gently dissolving away. Your total body is revitalized and fortified with powerful, rejuvenating energy. As the dynamic energy drawn from your inner fountain and the outer cosmic fountain blend and surge throughout your physical body, you can sense the warm restoration of youth and vigor.

Step 4. Conclusion. End the procedure by envisioning both your inner sparkling fountain of youth and the outer iridescent green cosmic fountain of youth. Bring your hands together as a gesture of your oneness with the two fountains and the powerful merging within yourself of inner and outer rejuvenating energy.

Day Five

Goal: The goal for day five of our plan is threefold: first, to acquire strategies that replenish your inner reservoir of rejuvenation resources; second, to generate and transfer cosmic energy to designated biological areas; and third, to protect the aura and prevent depletion of rejuvenating energy.

Day five introduces three strategies, each focusing on the self's aura energy system. Rejuvenation Replacement Therapy jumpstarts the total aura system and fortifies it with a powerful increase of new energy. The second strategy, Concentration and Transfer of Cosmic Energy, generates a visible concentration of pure cosmic energy and transfers it to specific body areas that may need energizing or renewal. The third strategy, the Finger Interlock Procedure, counteracts so-called psychic vampirism and restores lost energy. It energizes the aura and erects a sphere of protective energy that envelops the aura to temporarily shield it from further assault.

Rejuvenation Replacement Therapy

Step 1. Inner Aura Core. Settle back into a comfortable position, and with your eyes closed, envision your inner aura core as a glowing, pulsating orb with power to distribute energy throughout the aura enveloping your physical body.

Step 2. External Aura. Envision your external aura as a series of spheres within spheres of energy enveloping the physical body.

Step 3. Cosmic Energy System. Envision a cosmic core of limitless energy situated at the center of the universe, radiating energy in all directions to sustain and energize the total universe. Think of your own energy system with its core and surrounding energy as a replica of the cosmic energy system.

Step 4. Cosmic Congruency. Envision the outermost region of your aura system interfacing infinite energy of cosmic origin. Embrace the energy emanating from the center of the cosmos, and allow it to meld with your own energy system. Sense the integration of personal and cosmic energy, first in the external regions of your aura, and then throughout your total aura system.

Step 5. Energy Amplification. As your energy system interacts with the ultimate source of cosmic energy, sense the tremendous burst of rejuvenating cosmic energy in your aura's inner core, and then spreading progressively outward until your total aura is fully infused with new energy.

Concentration and Transfer of Cosmic Energy

Step 1. Goal Formulation. Formulate your goals, to include identifying the specific biological region, function, or system to be energized.

Step 2. Energy Concentration. Bring your palms together and rub them briskly against each other. Upon sensing the build-up of energy between your palms, slowly separate them, and with your hands cupped, notice the ball of pure white energy suspended between your palms.

Step 3. Energy Transfer. Place the ball of cosmic energy at any designated body location, and gently massage it into the aura by using circular motions while carefully avoiding direct contact with the physical body, which can negate the transfer effort by scattering the energy. To energize a particular physical organ or body region, gently massage the ball of energy into the aura at that location. To rejuvenate a biological system, such as the cardiovascular, or to stimulate the rejuvenation process, place the ball of energy at your solar plexus region and gently massage it into the aura. To erase the external signs of aging, place the ball of energy at the area to be rejuvenated and gently massage it into the aura, again using circular motions and carefully avoiding physical touch. You can even energize the brain with this procedure by placing the ball of energy anywhere around the head region and gently massaging it into the aura.

Step 4. Aura Balancing and Attunement. Balance your aura system by again rubbing your hands together briskly and then touching your temples with your fingertips as you affirm: *I am fully balanced and attuned, both inwardly and outwardly.*

Step 5. Rejuvenation Cue: Hand Rub-Temple Touch. Tell yourself in your own words that by simply rubbing your hands together and touching your temples, you can reactivate rejuvenation of both mind and body.

Finger Interlock Procedure

Step 1. Finger Interlock Gesture. Begin the procedure by joining the tips of the thumb and middle finger of each hand to form two circles. Next, bring your hands together to form interlocked circles. Hold the finger interlock position for the remainder of the procedure.

Step 2. Energy Protection. Envision a bright sphere of pure energy enveloping your total aura as a shield against any incoming force.

Step 3. Energy Infusion. With the protective sphere in place, sense your aura's innermost core pulsating with power and dispersing vibrant energy throughout your full aura. Let your total being—mind, body, and spirit— become fully infused and revitalized with radiant new energy.

Step 4. Affirmation. Affirm in your own words the empowering effects of the procedure. Examples are: *I am energized and fully enveloped in a protective shield or radiant energy. I am invigorated and fully infused with bright rejuvenating energy. I am protected, energized, and empowered!*

Step 5. Empowerment Cue. Affirm that by simply forming the interlock gesture, you can at any time instantly reactivate the energizing, rejuvenating effects of the procedure.

Day Six

Goal: The goal for day six is to acquire skill in using the quartz crystal and the pyramid as rejuvenation tools.

Day six introduces two strategies that introduce tangible objects as rejuvenation tools. The Crystal Rejuvenation Procedure guides selecting, programming, and applying the crystal for rejuvenation purposes. The second strategy, Pyramid of Youth, uses a small model of the Great Pyramid to promote rejuvenation and longevity. For this procedure, the pyramid can be of any material, but must be small enough to hold in the hand.

Crystal Rejuvenation Procedure

Step 1. Selecting a Crystal. In selecting an appropriate crystal from an assortment, mentally articulate your rejuvenation goals—arresting aging, becoming revitalized, looking younger, living longer, staying healthy, and so forth—as you pass your hand, palm side down, over the assortment. Notice individual crystals and sense their special energies. Eventually, a certain crystal will "stand out" from the others or seem to "call out" to you. Pick up the crystal and, gently cupping it in your hand, sense your interactions with it. A positive, harmonious interaction confirms the appropriateness of your choice. If you are in doubt, return the crystal to its place in the assortment, and repeat the above process. (Not infrequently, the crystal to be eventually selected is the particular crystal that commanded attention at the beginning of the viewing process.)

Step 2. Clearing the Crystal. To clear the crystal of any previous programming or extraneous energies, simply hold it under cool (not hot) running water for approximately one minute as you stroke it gently with your fingers. You will sense when the clearing process is complete. Place the deprogrammed crystal on a towel and let it air dry.

Step 3. Programming the Crystal. To program the crystal for rejuvenation purposes, hold it in your cupped hand and, with your eyes closed, state your rejuvenation goals. Form mental images of your goals and affirm them as positive expectations rather than some distant, nebulous possibility. For instance, you can picture yourself at your peak of youth with inner biological functions revitalized and all outer signs of aging erased. At this stage, be as imaginative and adventurous as you wish. Give your own energy system permission to interact with the energy system of the crystal. Sense the rejuvenating interaction as it occurs, and invite the crystal to continue to work with you as your partner. In your own words, affirm the reality of the rejuvenation process already initiated through your interaction with the crystal. Examples are: *The energies of youth are now flowing throughout my total being. Mentally, physically, and spiritually, I am renewed. An abundance of anti-aging energy is now at my command. My interaction with the crystal is a fountain of youth that cannot fail.* To complete the programming, address the crystal with the simple message, *Please stay*, which is usually sufficient to save the program.

Step 4. Using the Programmed Crystal. A programmed crystal works best when it is in close proximity to the person using it. Like programming the crystal, using the crystal for rejuvenation requires physical touch and conscious interaction. During your waking hours, either wearing the crystal as an ornament or carrying it in your pocket or purse is recommended. To unleash its rejuvenation capacities, periodically interact with the crystal by stroking it while envisioning your rejuvenation goals. During sleep, keep the crystal nearby and in full view, such as on a bedside table or dresser. Immediately before falling asleep, envision the crystal and sense your connection to it.

Pyramid of Youth

Step 1. Selecting the Pyramid. Select an appropriate pyramid model that can be conveniently held in the hand. Be careful to select a pyramid replica that is exactly proportional to the Great Pyramid.

Step 2. Pyramid Orientation. Placement of the pyramid, typically on a table, should facilitate a comfortable horizontal or slightly downward gaze. The direction orientation of the pyramid, so long as it rests on its base, does not seem to affect its rejuvenation potential.

Step 3. Pyramid Gazing. Gaze at the pyramid from a comfortable distance as you focus your full attention on it. Following a few moments of relaxed gazing, close your eyes and allow a clear image of the pyramid to emerge. Take plenty of time for the image to form in your mind, preferably as a bright pyramid against a dark background. If you have difficulty forming a mental image of the pyramid, repeat the gazing and imaging sequence until a clear image emerges. Once the image is clearly visible, center your full attention on it.

Step 4. Pyramid Arc of Light. With the pyramid image clearly visible in your mind, envision an arc of bright light connecting the apex of the external pyramid to the apex of your inner pyramid image.

Step 5. Rejuvenation Infusion. With the two pyramids—the one physical and the other mental—linked by the arc of light, envision the outer pyramid pulsating with energy that is, in turn, transferred to the inner pyramid through the arc of bright light. Visualize the inner pyramid, now totally energized, glowing with new power to revitalize every cell and fiber of your body. You can feel the opening of blocked channels and the vibrant flow of new energy. Envision your body now totally enveloped in a rejuvenating glow.

Step 6. Affirmation of Power. Affirm in your own words the rejuvenating effects of the procedure. Examples are: *I am now empowered to defy aging and defeat it. Vibrant new energy is now flowing throughout my total being. I am balanced and attuned to the inner and outer sources of rejuvenation.*

Step 7. Closing Infusion. Place the pyramid in the palm of your hand, and with your other hand held palm side down over the pyramid, sense again the powerful infusion of rejuvenating energy.

Step 8. Rejuvenation Cue. As the pyramid continues to rest between your palms, affirm that by holding the pyramid and visualizing the arc connecting it to your inner pyramid, you can instantly unleash abundant youth and health energies to flow throughout your total being.

Day Seven

Goal: The goal for day seven is twofold: first, to promote rejuvenating interactions with a selected tree; and second, to establish an energy vortex within yourself that can become your link to the highest cosmic source of rejuvenating energy.

For this final day of our seven-day plan, two new procedures are introduced. The Tree of Youth is a multifunctional strategy that centers on the tree as a powerhouse of energy. Through this strategy, you can increase the flow of positive energy by unblocking constricted energy channels, awaken dormant inner resources, access higher cosmic sources of rejuvenation, fortify your natural immunity against aging, and repair damaged or malfunctioning rejuvenating mechanisms. The second procedure, the Inner Vortex Strategy, generates a spiraling cone of energy over the body's solar plexus region. The apex of the vortex cone then becomes a powerful receptor of cosmic energy in its purest form.

Tree of Youth

Step 1. Selecting a Tree. The effectiveness of this procedure rests largely on selecting an appropriate tree. First, it is important to select a tree that appeals to you. Size, age, and type of tree are of only secondary importance. As in selecting a crystal, the tree that commands your attention or seems to beckon you is usually an excellent choice for this procedure. But as a rejuvenation resource, the tree must be more than visually appealing—it must be responsive to your touch. Place your palms against the tree's trunk, and sense its energies. Note the nature of your interaction with the tree and any spontaneous exchange of energies. Sense the compatibility of the two energy systems. Lift your hands a few inches from the tree and note the uninterrupted interaction between your hands and the tree.

Step 2. Naming the Tree. The purpose of this step is to personalize the tree you selected for the procedure by giving it a name. Remind yourself that the tree is an empowerment partner rather than simply a physical object. Think of it as a majestic creation of power and beauty. Then, with your palms still resting against the tree, close your eyes and assign the tree a name—any name that comes to mind. If you have difficulty naming the tree, use free association by simply saying "tree" and then allowing a name to emerge. (As an aside, many participants of this exercise discovered later on that the name they assigned the tree was the same as that of their ministering guide. This would suggest that personal guides are often spontaneous participants in tree interactions.)

Step 3. Tree Interaction. Although your interaction with the tree actually began with the selection process, it intensifies at this step and finally culminates in a powerful release of rejuvenating energy. As your palms continue to rest lightly against the tree, address it as your rejuvenation partner, calling it by its assigned name. Invite it, in your own words, to interact with you and share its rejuvenating powers. Take a few moments to sense the powerful frequencies of its energies melding with your own energies. Let the tree become an integral part of your own energy system. Sense the powerful transfer of the tree's energy, transforming and rejuvenating your own energy system. Let the tree's rejuvenating energy fully infuse your total being— mentally, physically, and spiritually. Think of the tree as the earth's antenna and your link to the cosmic source of all life. Let yourself become fully attuned to that limitless source of cosmic power.

Step 4. Disengagement. Slowly lift your palms, and while holding them a few inches from the tree, note the continuation of powerful energy infusion. Sense the harmony of the interaction and the wondrous energy resonating throughout your body.

Step 5. Conclusion. Address the tree, and in your own words, express your appreciation for its responsiveness to your rejuvenation needs. Finally, rest your palms again upon the tree and sense its magnificent power. At this point, you may experience a deep and enduring connection to the tree as not only a living system of great power, but also a supportive partner in your quest for rejuvenation.

Inner Vortex Strategy

Step 1. Goal Statement. State your intent to establish an energy vortex within yourself. Specify the empowerment functions of the vortex, such as rejuvenation and longevity or any other personal empowerment goal.

Step 2. Vortex Cone. While lying down and with your eyes closed, envision your solar plexus region as an abundant repository of bright energy. Using either hand, initiate circular clockwise motions a few inches from your body at your solar plexus region. Envision energy from your solar plexus becoming activated to spin clockwise, thus establishing a base for the vortex. Continue the clockwise motions using your hand's circular motions to form a spiraling cone of luminous energy rising from your body, with the solar plexus constituting the vortex's energizing base.

Step 3. Cosmic Infusion. With the spiraling cone of energy rising above your solar plexus, envision a bright beam of radiant energy connecting the apex of the vortex cone to the distant cosmic core of pure energy. Sense powerful energy infusing the vortex and then spreading throughout your body. Note the balancing, rejuvenating effect of the experience.

Step 4. Concluding Affirmation. Conclude the procedure with self-affirmations related to your goals as stated in Step 1. Examples are: *I am at my peak of personal power. The energies of my being are attuned to the cosmic source of my existence. I am at one with the cosmos.*

Summary

The seven-day plan now complete, you have established a strong foundation for rejuvenation. Rather than aging, even as you read this, you are well on your way to a younger, longer, and better life. The Fountain beckons—"wrinkledom" is no longer your destination. Equipped with the forty-five strategies presented in this book, you have all the resources you need for complete success. Living younger, longer, and better is now your destiny.

Chapter 11

Conclusion

As we go forward into the new millennium, living younger, longer, and better is one of our greatest personal challenges. Given what we already know, along with new knowledge poised at the edge of discovery, it is clear that the so-called "fixed" life span is not fixed at all. Whatever your age now, you can control the deterioration of aging so that your body does not self-destruct. It is conceivable, in fact, that you could live throughout the new century, if not beyond.

But merely living longer does not guarantee a better life. Most of us would prefer a brief life span with quality to a long life span without it. That's why quality of life is a major focus throughout this book. It is the "living better" component woven into each rejuvenation strategy. Also found throughout this book is a strong belief in our capacity for continuous growth and change. We are never too old or too young to learn new and better ways of living. Only by embracing change can we develop our potentials for a longer and richer life.

Flexibility is a critical component of any rejuvenation effort. Although the forty-five strategies presented in this book are organized into steps, they are not written into stone. They can be revised as needed to fit your own personal interests and preferences. Many of the strategies include rejuvenation cues designed for use independent of the full procedure to instantly activate the rejuvenation process. Examples are the toe lift, hand rub and temple touch, finger interlock, and praying hands, to mention but a few. Like the full procedures, cues are flexible—they can be altered or revised to include the substitution of other cues.

Only through recognizing the vast repository of inner and outer rejuvenating energy can we achieve our rejuvenation goals. Throughout this book, we steadfastly rejected all enfeebling cultural stereotypes and constricted conventional views of self-styled "authorities" that place limits on our capacity for rejuvenation. Within each of us is a receptive fountain of bountiful youth just waiting to be activated. Beyond that, the highest cosmic fountain of youth invites our interaction. Given these inner and outer resources, we have access to a limitless supply of healthful, rejuvenating energy.

The cosmic aspects of rejuvenation are too often overlooked in our search for the Fountain. Aside from directly tapping into higher cosmic planes and dimensions as sources of rejuvenating energy, we can enrich our rejuvenation efforts by getting to know our personal guides, cosmic teachers, and guardian angels. They are our personal contacts to the cosmic realm as well as direct sources of rejuvenating power. Getting to know them automatically enriches our lives. In the good times and the bad, they are there to share, guide, and protect. All it takes is a receptive mind to experience the wondrous power of their presence.

Awareness of our existence as an infinite life force is itself rejuvenating. Our destiny as conscious beings is abundant, endless life, not desolation and nothingness. When we cross over to the other side, personal identity and conscious awareness remain intact. Furthermore, at the moment of our transition, we are instantly transformed to the highest peaks of all our past growth. Even more important, all the resources we need for our continued growth and fulfillment remain available to us upon our entrance to that bright dimension.

Fortunately, all the elusive riches of the cosmic realm are within our reach in the here and now. At last, we have the required strategies and the essential resources to maximize our potentials for living a younger, longer, and better life.

Glossary

ageism. A common cultural stereotype in which age is seen as a downward shift in status and recognition.

age regression. A hypnosis procedure designed to explore past experiences which occurred in one's present lifetime but unavailable to conscious awareness.

Awakening Rejuvenation. A procedure designed to arrest the normal awakening state in order to access various inner rejuvenation resources.

Amethyst Amplification Procedure. A procedure which uses the amethyst gem to integrate inner and outer energy sources and balance them to produce an integrated state of renewal.

Astral Plane Procedure. An out-of-body strategy designed to access pure astral energy and transfer it to the physical body.

astral projection. A state of awareness in which the locus of perception shifts to result in a conscious sense of being in a spatial location outside or away from the physical body. Also known as out-of-body experience (OBE) and soul travel.

Astral Rejuvenation Through Hand Levitation. An procedure designed to rejuvenate the astral body and its physically body counterpart during the out-of-body state.

aura. A colorful energy enveloping the physical body. The aura is believed to be an external energy phenomenon emanating from an inner energy core which is linked to the cosmic source of our existence.

Aura Attunement Strategy. A procedure designed to bring the aura's multiple functions into a state of total oneness.

Aura Caress. A technique that identifies disruptions in the aura's frequency patterns, and classifies the aura's current level of attunement within a range of one to seven.

Aura Conditioning Strategy. A procedure designed for exercising the aura by generating a rhythmic pattern of aura expansion and contraction.

aura core. The indestructible center of energy believed to be situated in the body's solar plexus. The aura core is believed to be our connection to the infinite power of the universe.

Aura Hand-viewing Strategy. A structured procedure designed for self-viewing of the aura surrounding the hand.

Aura Rejuvenation Strategy. A procedure used to stimulate the aura's rejuvenation functions.

Balance and Attunement Strategy. A strategy designed first, to produced a balanced and attuned state in which mind, body, and spirit interact in complete harmony, and second, to tap outer cosmic sources of rejuvenating energy.

Concentration and Transfer of Cosmic Energy. A procedure that generates a visible concentration of energy and transfers it to a specific body area that may need energizing or renewal.

Control Center Strategy. A rejuvenation procedure designed to relax the physical body and introduce certain cognitive activities that slow the aging process and reverse the biological effects of aging.

cosmic congruency. A state in which the human aura system melds with energy emanating from the center of the cosmos.

Cosmic Fountain of Youth. A procedure that guides astral travel to the cosmic fountain of youth where the astral body is bathed in rejuvenating energy.

Cosmic Infusion Procedure. A procedure designed to tap the higher cosmic source of rejuvenation energy.

Cosmic Interaction Strategy. A procedure structured to access cosmic rejuvenation specialists and transfer rejuvenating energy of cosmic origin to the physical body.

Crystal Rejuvenation Procedure. A procedure designed as a guide for selecting, programming, and applying the crystal as a rejuvenation tool.

Destination Travel. An out-of-body procedure designed to generate a positive, optimistic state of mind while inducing a tranquil, relaxed state.

Discarnate State Regression. A hypnosis procedure that focuses on either our existence before our first incarnation or our existence between our past lives.

Dream of Youth. A presleep strategy that generates rejuvenating images that are transferred to the subconscious where they activate dormant rejuvenation potentials.

duality principle. The concept that our basic makeup consists of both a biological body and a nonbiological counterpart.

Emerald Cord Procedure. A strategy designed to access the emerald cosmic plane and transport its healthful, rejuvenating energy to the physical body during the out-of-body state.

Emerald Pool Strategy. A procedure using the emerald to promote rejuvenation by flooding the mind and body with youthful energy.

Emerald Ray Procedure. A procedure that introduces imagery of an emerald ray of light connecting the emerald to the third-eye region and then to the brain in an effort to awaken the brain's renewal potentials and stimulate rejuvenation.

Finger Interlock Procedure. A procedure to protect against psychic vampirism by joining the fingers to form interlocking circles.

Fingertip Engagement Procedure. A procedure that uses fingertip-to-fingertip touch to reduce stress, induce a state of inner harmony, and activate rejuvenation.

Hand-Clasp Strategy. An assertive procedure designed to induce a state of physical tension in order to generate mental and physical balance.

Higher Plane Rejuvenation. A procedure designed to facilitate interaction with the green cosmic plane in order to revitalize and renew the physical body.

hypnoproduction. The emergence, typically spontaneous, of full-blown potentials during the trance state. Examples are fluency in a new language or advanced knowledge of a new discipline.

hypnosis. An altered state of awareness in which our subconscious faculties and resources become increasingly responsive to conscious probes.

hypnotic regression. A hypnosis procedure that explores past experiences, including current lifetime experiences buried in the subconscious as well as past lives.

Hypnotic Rejuvenation Through Hand Levitation. A rejuvenation procedure which uses the hand levitation induction technique to establish a rejuvenation link between the mind and body.

Inner-balance and Attunement Strategy. A procedure that focuses on the interaction between the mind and body in order to induce a state of attunement and balance within the self.

Inner Vortex Strategy. A procedure designed to establish an energy vortex within the self, which, in turn, becomes our link to the highest cosmic source of pure energy.

Interdimensional Tabling. A procedure in which a small table is used as an interdimensional tool to access discarnate sources of rejuvenation.

internal locus of control. The inner ability to control your own life and the forces that influence it.

Nature Walk. A procedure that focuses on the powerful elements of nature and our capacity to use them as rejuvenation resources.

negative stress. Corrosive energy that asserts a wear-and-tear effect on both the mind and body.

out-of-body experience (OBE). See *astral projection.*

past-life regression. A hypnosis strategy that uncovers experiences of past incarnations, as well as existence before one's first incarnation along with experiences in the discarnate realm between incarnations.

Pearl of Youth. A procedure in which the pearl is used to counteract the effects of aging.

Pk. See *psychokinesis.*

positive stress. Constructive energy that is potentially empowering both mentally and physically.

posthypnotic cue. Typically a gesture, thought, or mental image which is executed at will following the trance state to activate certain designated effects of hypnosis.

postprocedure cue. Typically a gesture, thought, or mental image which is executed at will following a procedure to activate certain designated effects.

Progressive Imagery Formula. A strategy designed specifically to build basic imagery skills and apply them toward stress management and rejuvenation.

psychic vampire. The individual whose energy system is flawed and thus sustained only by the habitual consumption of energy from other human energy systems.

psychic vampirism. A complex, interrelated phenomenon in which one's own energies are transferred to the psychic vampire whose strategies are mental instead of physical. See *psychic vampire*.

psychokinesis (Pk). The capacity of the mind to influence external conditions independent of physical contact or intermediate instrumentation.

Rejuvenation Replacement Therapy. A self-intervention strategy designed to replenish the inner reservoir of rejuvenation resources by generating a state of cosmic congruency.

Pyramid of Youth. A procedure using a small model of the Great Pyramid to promote rejuvenation and longevity.

Rejuvenation Through Age Regression. A hypnosis procedure designed to create a peak infusion and continuous flow of rejuvenation for persons who are beyond their peaks of youth and vitality.

Rejuvenation Through Past-Life Regression. A hypnosis procedure designed to select potentially rejuvenating past-life experiences and convey them to conscious awareness in an effort to activate a rejuvenation interaction.

Sapphire of Youth. A step-by-step procedure that used the sapphire to initiate a balanced, internal flow of anti-aging energy.

self-hypnosis. A trance state that is self-induced and self-managed independent of a trained hypnotist.

Sleep Anti-aging Strategy. A procedure designed to manipulate sleep and redirect it in an effort to awaken dormant age-defying functions.

Sleep Enrichment Strategy. Implemented just prior to falling asleep, the procedure is designed to energize the subconscious and awaken a variety of dormant anti-aging mechanisms.

Super Cosmic Highway. An out-of-body procedure that facilitates an empowering interaction with the cosmic realm as the highest source of rejuvenating energy.

table tapping. An interactive procedure in which a small table is used to "tap into" the discarnate realm and its wealth of empowerment resources. Also known as table tilting.

table tilting. See table tapping.

telepathy. Mind-to-mind communication.

Toe-lift Technique. A rejuvenation procedure designed to induce a deeply relaxed state, extinguish negative stress, and saturate the body's multiple systems with rejuvenating energy.

Tree of Youth. A procedure designed to promote rejuvenating interactions with a selected tree.

vortex. So-called "power spots" in which energies from multiple sources create a synergistic interaction.

Vortex Interactive Strategy. A procedure structured to initiate a rejuvenating vortex interaction and to target positive vortex energies to designated goals.

X Formation. A gesture in which the arms are crossed over the chest to generate a state of inner balance.

Suggested Reading

Ajzen, L. and M. Fishbein. *Understanding Attitudes and Predicting Social Behavior.* Englewood Cliffs, N.J.: Prentice Hall. 1980.

Baltes, M. M. *The Many Faces of Dependency in Old Age.* New York: Cambridge University Press. 1996.

Crowne, P. A. *Cardiovascular Psychophysiology: A Perspective.* New York: Plenum. 1981.

Cumes, David. *The Spirit of Healing.* St. Paul, Minn.: Llewellyn Publications. 1999.

Erdelys, M. H. *The Recovery of Unconscious Memories.* Chicago: University of Chicago Press. 1996.

Freedy, J. R. and S. E. Hobfall, eds. *Traumatic Stress.* New York: Plenum. 1995.

Finley, Guy. *Design Your Destiny: Shape your Future in 12 Easy Steps.* St. Paul, Minn.: Llewellyn Publications. 1999.

Jacobs, R. H. *Be an Outrageous Older Woman.* New York: Harper-Collins. 1997.

Kalton, G. *Introduction to Survey Sampling*. Newbury Park, Calif.: Sage Publications. 1983.

Klein, W. C. and M. Bloom. *Successful Aging: Strategies for Healthy Living*. New York: Plenum. 1997.

Loehle, C. *Thinking Strategically*. New York: Cambridge University Press. 1996.

Neugarten, B. L. *The Meanings of Age*. Chicago: University of Chicago Press. 1996.

Nucho, A. O. *Spontaneous Creative Imagery: Problem Solving and Life Enhancing Skills*. Springfield, Ill.: Thomas. 1995.

———. *Stress Management: The Quest for Zest*. Springfield, Ill.: Thomas. 1988.

Ogilvie, R. and J. Harsh, eds. *Sleep Onset: Normal and Abnormal Processes*. Washington, D.C.: American Psychological Association. 1994.

Ornstein, R. *The Evolution of Consciousness*. Englewood Cliffs, N.J.: Prentice Hall. 1992.

Paulson, Genevieve Lewis. *Energy-Focused Meditation: Body, Mind, Spirit*. St. Paul, Minn.: Llewellyn Publications. 1999.

Rieber, R. W. *Manufacturing Stress: Psychopathy in Everyday Life*. New York: Plenum. 1997.

Rose, N. *Inventing Ourselves*. New York: Cambridge University Press. 1996.

Segal, N. L., G. E. Weisfeld, and C. C. Wisefeld, eds. *Uniting Psychology and Biology*. Washington, D.C.: American Psychological Association. 1997.

Slate, Joe H. *Aura Energy for Health, Healing & Balance*. St. Paul, Minn.: Llewellyn Publications. 1999.

———. *Astral Projection and Psychic Empowerment: Techniques for Mastering the Out-of-Body Experience*. St. Paul, Minn.: Llewellyn Publications. 1998.

———. *Psychic Empowerment for Health and Fitness.* St. Paul, Minn.: Llewellyn Publications. 1996.

———. *Psychic Empowerment: A 7-Day Plan for Self Development.* St. Paul, Minn.: Llewellyn Publications. 1995.

Welch, Pamela. *The Energy Body Connection: The Healing Experience of Self-Embodiment.* St. Paul, Minn.: Llewellyn Publications. 1999.

Wilson, Colin. *After Life; Survival of the Soul.* St. Paul, Minn.: Llewellyn Publications. 1999.

Young, G. D. *Adult Development, Therapy, and Culture: A Postmodern Synthesis.* New York: Plenum. 1997.

Index

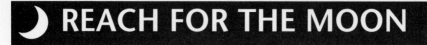

REACH FOR THE MOON

Llewellyn publishes hundreds of books on your favorite subjects! To get these exciting books, including the ones on the following pages, check your local bookstore or order them directly from Llewellyn.

ORDER BY PHONE

- Call toll-free within the U.S. and Canada, 1-800-THE MOON
- In Minnesota, call (651) 291-1970
- We accept VISA, MasterCard, and American Express

ORDER BY MAIL

- Send the full price of your order (MN residents add 7% sales tax) in U.S. funds, plus postage & handling to:

  Llewellyn Worldwide
  P.O. Box 64383, Dept. 1-56718-633-5
  St. Paul, MN 55164–0383, U.S.A.

POSTAGE & HANDLING

(For the U.S., Canada, and Mexico)

- $4.00 for orders $15.00 and under
- $5.00 for orders over $15.00
- No charge for orders over $100.00

We ship UPS in the continental United States. We ship standard mail to P.O. boxes. Orders shipped to Alaska, Hawaii, The Virgin Islands, and Puerto Rico are sent first-class mail. Orders shipped to Canada and Mexico are sent surface mail.

International orders: Airmail—add freight equal to price of each book to the total price of order, plus $5.00 for each non-book item (audio tapes, etc.).

Surface mail—Add $1.00 per item.

Allow 2 weeks for delivery on all orders.
Postage and handling rates subject to change.

DISCOUNTS

We offer a 20% discount to group leaders or agents. You must order a minimum of 5 copies of the same book to get our special quantity price.

FREE CATALOG

Get a free copy of our color catalog, *New Worlds of Mind and Spirit.* Subscribe for just $10.00 in the United States and Canada ($30.00 overseas, airmail). Many bookstores carry *New Worlds*— ask for it!

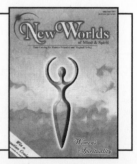

Visit our web site at www.llewellyn.com for more information.

Aura Energy for Health, Healing & Balance

Joe H. Slate, Ph.D.

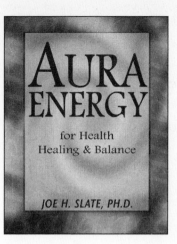

Imagine an advanced energy/information system that contains the chronicle of your life—past, present, and future. By referring to it, you could discover exciting new dimensions to your existence. You could uncover important resources for new insights, growth, and power.

You possess such a system *right now.* It is your personal aura. In his latest book, Dr. Joe H. Slate illustrates how each one of us has the power to see the aura, interpret it, and fine-tune it to promote mental, physical, and spiritual well-being. College students have used his techniques to raise their grade-point averages, gain admission to graduate programs, and eventually get the jobs they want. Now you can use his aura empowerment program to initiate an exciting new spiral of growth in all areas of your life.

1-56718-637-8, 288 pp., 6 x 9 in.   **$12.95**

*Astral Projection
and Psychic
Empowerment*

Joe H. Slate, Ph.D.

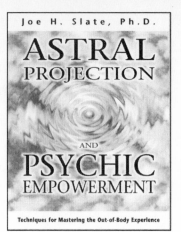

There is probably no other human phenomenon so steeped in mystery yet so potentially empowering as the out-of-body experience (OBE). To experience this remarkable phenomenon is to discover new meaning to our existence as a conscious, enduring energy force in the universe.

This book presents a wide range of new techniques designed to maximize, and in some cases, exceed the limits of your mind's powers. It explores the underlying nature of OBEs, including several controlled laboratory studies, and develops an innovative OBE technology consisting of sound principles and step-by-step procedures. Finally, this book presents you with a seven-day plan to unleash your highest growth potentials. Beginning with simple practice and conditioning exercises, the plan progresses to more complex strategies, and finally culminates in OBE travel to the highest realms of cosmic power.

1-56718-636-X, 240 pp., 6 x 9 in., illus. $12.95

To order, call 1-800-THE MOON
Prices subject to change without notice

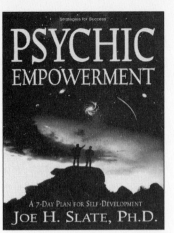

Psychic Empowerment

Joe H. Slate, Ph.D.

Use 100% of your mind power in just one week! You've heard it before: each of us is filled with an abundance of untapped power—yet we only use one-tenth of its potential. Now a clinical psychologist and famed researcher in parapsychology shows you how to probe your mind's psychic faculties and manifest your capacity to access the higher planes of the mind.

The psychic experience validates your true nature and connects you to your inner knowing. Dr. Slate reveals the life-changing nature of psychic phenomena—including telepathy, out-of-body experiences, and automatic writing. At the same time, he shows you how to develop a host of psychic abilities including psychokinesis, crystal gazing, and table tilting.

The final section of the book outlines his accelerated *7-Day Psychic Development Plan* through which you can unleash your innate power and wisdom without further delay.

1-56718-635-1, 256 pp., 6 x 9 in.   **$12.95**

To order, call 1-800-THE MOON
Prices subject to change without notice

Your Health

It's a Question of Balance

**Dr. Igor Cetojevic
with Francesca Pinoni**

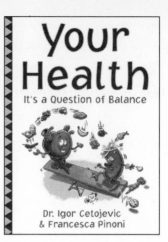

If you're one of the growing number of people beginning to look into alternative therapies, then this quick-reading introduction to Chinese medicine, electromagnetic vibrations, and the use of gemstones in healing is just what the doctor ordered—Dr. Cetojevic, that is, who explains it all in terms even a child can understand.

Trained in both Western and Eastern medicine, Dr. Cetojevic shows you how to improve your health by following the principles of Yin (cold, dark) and Yang (hot, light) to tailor your diet and lifestyle to your individual constitution. See how your body's organs correlate with the time of day and seasons of the year, and how you can use that knowledge to improve your own health and well-being.

Your Health is full of practical advice you can use immediately, including how to use a quartz crystal to make wine taste better and eliminate hangovers, and how to improve your sleep just by moving your bed!

1-56718-121-X, 192 pp., 5 ³/₁₆ x 8 in., 41 illus.   **$12.95**

To order, call 1-800-THE MOON
Prices subject to change without notice

Chakras, Auras, and the New Spirituality

Genevieve Lewis Paulson & Stephen J. Paulson

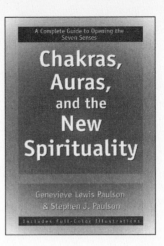

The numbers seven and twelve permeate our lives: there are seven days in a week, twelve months in a year, and seven notes in a scale (twelve if you include the sharps). Kundalini (evolutionary energy) starts with seven main chakras.

This book explores the spiritual rhythm of these two numbers, and how by opening up to their energies through meditation you can speed up your personal growth. Discover the seven bodies of the human constitution, and the seven corresponding planes of evolution—from primitive to cosmic consciousness. Learn about our seven senses, and practice meditation exercises to lift your consciousness to a greater level. Develop your seven eyes and your seven brains for clearer vision and and greater creativity. Finally, peek into the seven other realities, including the Akashic records and parallel dimensions, and discover the little-known system of the seven spheres, first introduced by Israel Regardie.

1-56718-513-4, 312 pp., 6 x 9 in., full-color 8-pp. insert

$17.95

Energy-Focused Meditation
Body • Mind • Spirit

Genevieve Lewis Paulson

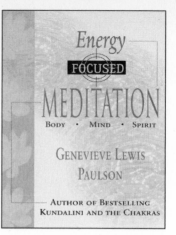

Meditation has many purposes: healing, past life awareness, balance, mental clarity, and relaxation. It is a way of opening into areas that are beyond your normal thinking patterns. In fact, what we now call "altered states" and "peak experiences"—tremendous experiences of transcendental states—can become normal occurrences when you know how to contact the higher energy vibrations.

Most people think that peak experiences happen, at best, only a few times in life. Through meditation, however, it is possible to develop your higher awareness so you can bring more peak happenings about by concentrated effort. *Energy Focused Meditation* is full of techniques for those who wish to claim those higher vibrations and expanded awareness for their lives today.

1-56718-512-6, 224 pp., 6 x 9 in., 17 illus.   **$12.95**